TAKE CONTROL OF YOUR DRINKING

SECOND EDITION

Take Control

of

Your Drinking

A PRACTICAL GUIDE TO
Alcohol Moderation, Sobriety, and
When to Get Professional Help

Michael S. Levy

JOHNS HOPKINS UNIVERSITY PRESS

Baltimore

Note to the Reader: This book is not meant to substitute for medical care of people who have depression or other mental disorders, and treatment should not be based solely on its contents. Instead, treatment must be developed in a dialogue between the individual and his or her physician. My book has been written to help with that dialogue.

Drug dosage: The author and publisher have made reasonable efforts to determine that the selection of drugs discussed in this text conform to the practices of the general medical community. The medications described do not necessarily have specific approval by the US Food and Drug Administration for use in the diseases for which they are recommended. In view of ongoing research, changes in governmental regulation, and the constant flow of information relating to drug therapy and drug reactions, the reader is urged to check the package insert of each drug for any change in indications and dosage and for warnings and precautions. This is particularly important when the recommended agent is a new and/or infrequently used drug.

© 2007, 2021 Johns Hopkins University Press
All rights reserved. Published 2021
Printed in the United States of America on acid-free paper
9 8 7 6 5 4 3 2 1

Johns Hopkins University Press
2715 North Charles Street
Baltimore, Maryland 21218-4363
www.press.jhu.edu

Library of Congress Cataloging-in-Publication Data

Names: Levy, Michael S., 1953– author.
Title: Take control of your drinking : a practical guide to alcohol moderation, sobriety,
    and when to get professional help / Michael S. Levy.
Description: Second edition. | Baltimore : Johns Hopkins University Press, 2021.
    | Revised edition of: Take control of your drinking—and you may not need to quit.
    2007. | Includes bibliographical references and index.
Identifiers: LCCN 2020009000 | ISBN 9781421439433 (hardcover) | ISBN 9781421439440
    (paperback) | ISBN 9781421439457 (ebook)
Subjects: LCSH: Drinking of alcoholic beverages. | Temperance. | Alcoholism—Treatment.
Classification: LCC HV5035 .L48 2021 | DDC 613.81—dc23
LC record available at https://lccn.loc.gov/2020009000

A catalog record for this book is available from the British Library.

Special discounts are available for bulk purchases of this book. For more information, please contact Special Sales at specialsales@press.jhu.edu.

Johns Hopkins University Press uses environmentally friendly book materials, including recycled text paper that is composed of at least 30 percent post-consumer waste, whenever possible.

Contents

TAKE CONTROL OF YOUR DRINKING

Introduction

About 30 years ago, I started working with people who were hurting themselves by drinking too much. At that time, the three most important principles I was taught were (1) people *had* to admit that they had the disease of *alcoholism*; (2) people *had* to stop drinking entirely; and (3) people *had* to get treatment if they were going to stop alcohol from ruining their lives. And treatment in most every case meant going to Alcoholics Anonymous (AA) meetings because AA was the only approach believed to work. If people wouldn't admit they had a disease, or they refused to stop drinking, or they simply wouldn't go to AA meetings, this was a sign of their *denial*, or their unwillingness to admit they had a drinking problem. This thinking still persists in some circles today.

The AA expression "Keep it simple, stupid" applied not only to the alcoholic but also to the professional who was treating the alcoholic. Don't do anything fancy or different—just get the alcoholic to admit that he or she is an alcoholic, get the person to stop drinking, and get the person to go to "90 meetings in 90 days."

I was even told that I shouldn't treat alcoholics with psychotherapy. Exploring how drinking may have something to do with patients' emotional life conflicted with the idea that their problem with alcohol was a primary disease that had nothing to do with anything else, especially their psychological life. The message I received was that seeing alcoholics in therapy instead of insisting they go to AA meetings would simply increase their denial and foster the idea that they didn't have a disease.

Unfortunately, I found that many people resisted one or more of these well-intended suggestions. Some reported that they had checked

1

out the AA scene, but it just wasn't for them. They told me that instead of going to meetings, they preferred to spend their time doing something more fun than listening to alcoholics talk about their problems. Some even said that they hated AA meetings. Their reasons included not liking the spiritual overtones in AA meetings and not liking the rigid approach often recommended in AA. Sometimes they told me that AA meetings made them feel more unhappy when they heard such painful and depressing life stories. Others seemed to be private people who didn't like the public exposure of going to meetings. And others even told me that going to meetings made them want to drink more. Rather than hearing all of the talk about drinking and the problems drinking caused, these people wanted to put their alcohol problems behind them and not be constantly reminded of them.

What was most interesting to me was that many of these people admitted that they had an alcohol problem, and they didn't seem to be *in denial*. They just didn't like going to meetings. They preferred working with a therapist on an individual basis. What was I to do? Refuse to see them, or should I work with them in the manner they wanted? And what if I continued to see them, and they continued to drink? Was I doing them a disservice by seeing them in therapy? Was I making things worse and giving them the wrong care?

There were some people who refused to admit that they had the disease of *alcoholism*. They told me that they didn't like being labeled an *alcoholic*. This label made them feel as though something was terribly wrong with them. On the other hand, they could admit that they had a drinking problem, and they acknowledged that they often drank too much. Some viewed their problem with alcohol simply as a bad habit that they had learned over time.

In my opinion, many of these people weren't in denial. Although refusing to acknowledge the idea that they were alcoholics was, for some, a way to minimize their problem, for others this was not true. Many knew that they had to do something about their drinking and that drinking was clearly a problem for them. They just didn't like being labeled an alcoholic. This forced me to question how important it was for people with a drinking problem to admit they had the disease of alcoholism. Wasn't it fine for people to view their alcohol problem however they wished? Wasn't it more important for people to develop a plan to address their drinking than to get them to believe a particular concept? Who cares what they call their problem? More important is that they do something about it.

I worked with some people who wanted to try to moderate or control their drinking instead of choosing to become abstinent. I was totally unprepared for this, as everything I had learned told me that people needed to stop drinking completely in order to get better. In fact, I had learned that the wish to moderate one's drinking was the most blatant form of denial because it represented a refusal to acknowledge powerlessness over alcohol consumption. The whole notion of alcoholism is that people cannot moderate their drinking and must become abstinent to get better. Trying to control drinking was a clear sign: these people were not admitting they had a drinking problem, and they were still in denial.

What was I to do in this circumstance? Confront them about their denial and their unwillingness to do what it takes to get better? Should I tell them that their wish to moderate their drinking is just that—a wish—and that trying to control problem drinking simply isn't possible? I certainly didn't want to do anything that would further their denial. Or should I work with them on their goal to moderate their drinking? Maybe I needed to do this as a way to engage them in the treatment process. Even if it weren't possible to control their drinking, perhaps they needed to try it and fail so they could figure out that moderating drinking *wasn't* possible for them.

I was in a quandary. First, I was concerned that I'd be viewed as a quack if I worked with people to help them moderate their drinking. I might be laughed at, and my stature as a psychologist who knew something about alcohol problems might be diminished. I was also concerned about my professional liability if people didn't get better and drinking continued to cause them harm. Maybe I would be held legally liable if their continued drinking hurt them.

At the same time, I was beginning to see that the "one size fits all" approach simply didn't work and that if I was going to be successful, people needed to be given the freedom to make their own decisions. If people first wanted to try to moderate their drinking, perhaps they should be given this choice. And again, maybe they needed to discover whether controlling their drinking was possible before they would consider abstaining from alcohol completely.

Fortunately, I had some supervisors with a flexible approach who gave me the freedom and permission to work with people in less traditional ways. I am reminded of a conversation I had with one of my supervisors early on in my training. I told him that I was seeing some people with alcohol problems in my private practice who continued to drink and who refused to admit that they were alcoholic. They also refused to make full use of AA meetings in the community. I wondered whether I should continue to see them or whether I should terminate therapy, as they weren't entirely ready for treatment. My inclination was to continue to work with them, but I questioned that stance given what I had learned. What my supervisor said to me was that I would have an extremely small practice if I only saw people who admitted they were alcoholics, who went to AA meetings consistently, and who never drank. I would also be limiting myself to the easiest of patients.

I was discovering that different things worked with different people and that individuals *must be allowed to find out for themselves what they need to do to get their lives in order.* I knew this from my general clinical training, and I simply started to apply this thinking to the treatment of people who struggled with alcohol. As straightforward as this idea may seem, it was revolutionary at the time.

As my confidence grew and I gained more experience in the treatment of drinking problems, I began to see that no two people who struggled with alcohol consumption were the same. While some had serious problems with alcohol and clearly needed to stop drinking to avoid destroying their lives, others seemed to get by for years, though they drank problematically, and their lives didn't seem to get worse and worse and worse. Others had a pattern of not drinking for long periods of time, interspersed with brief periods of heavy drinking. I also saw some adolescents and young adults who struggled with alcohol but who seemed to mature out of their difficulties essentially on their own.

And my instinct that different approaches worked for different people was confirmed. For some, AA was a godsend; for others, it provided no benefit. And some people obtained help from other types of self-help meetings. For many people, abstinence was the only route to recovery; others learned to moderate their drinking. I also discovered that many people stopped alcohol from ruining their life without outside help of any kind, or through an extremely limited contact with treatment. They just seemed to make up their mind to change their life and their relationship to alcohol. I also got the opportunity to meet some people who had been in and out of the treatment system for years because of heavy drinking and who seemed as though they would never stop drinking and get their lives together. Then, at some point, something seemed to click, and they were able to stop drinking. Treatment appeared to be almost the *least* important factor in this; what seemed most important was their *internal motivation and desire to change.*

I am reminded of Nancy, a woman I worked with who ran a shelter program and who years earlier had been in and out of hospitals numerous times because of her out-of-control drinking. When I met her, she had been abstinent from alcohol for about 10 years. I was early in my career, and I wanted to learn more about drinking problems and how people were finally able to resolve their problem with alcohol. I decided to ask her what did it for her and what factors she believed enabled her to stop drinking. Was there some event in her life or some type of treatment that finally helped her achieve success? She thought about my question for a while and then simply stated, "I guess I was ready."

Answers like this surprised me because I had been taught that treatment was essential and that if left untreated, alcoholism was a chronic, progressive, and fatal disease. I had learned that the saying "the man takes a drink, the drink takes a drink, and the drink takes the man" applied to everyone. In order to avoid a mental hospital, jail, or death, a person diagnosed with alcoholism had no choice but to get treatment and to stop drinking altogether. I came to realize that this was not entirely true.

After working in this field for many years and refining how I worked with people, I decided to write a book for people who struggle in some way with alcohol. In this book I would explain my thinking about alcohol problems and my approach to treatment. I decided to do this for three main reasons. First, there is considerable misunderstanding about the nature and treatment of alcohol problems that I want to dispel. Having an alcohol problem is now an "out of the closet" subject, and many people know something about it. As the saying goes, "a little knowledge is dangerous," and I want to give people *more* knowledge so that they are better informed. People who are affected by an alcohol problem and those who love them should have this knowledge and should not be misinformed.

Second, I wanted to write a book that offers people an approach they can use to *help themselves* with a drinking problem regardless of how they choose to understand or address it. In fact, I wanted to write a book that gives people total control and complete freedom over how they choose to perceive and handle their problem. People should not be forced to believe a certain idea or be told what to do to resolve a drinking problem. They should be free to understand their problem with alcohol in any way they want. They should also be free to discover what they need to do in order to stop alcohol from ruining their life.

Third, it became obvious to me that many, many people do not seek and do not want treatment for their alcohol problem. There are many reasons why people do not get outside help. They may be too ashamed to ask for help, or they may simply be private people who do not like sharing the intimate aspects of their life with strangers. Some people prefer to do things on their own and don't like having to rely on others. And some, while concerned about their drinking, believe that going to treatment means they will have to stop drinking, which they are not ready to do. Providing a resource that allows people to help themselves on their own was another reason I wrote this book.

The first edition of this book came out in 2007, and I was delighted when I was asked to write a second edition. From the time when the book was first printed until now, my thinking has continued to expand and evolve. Throughout the book, I have added new information, tools, and things to think about that will help people resolve their drinking problem. During this time, there also have been some changes in our understanding and treatment of drinking problems, as well as some important shifts in the treatment field, and I have included these new ideas in this edition.

Helping people try to moderate their use of alcohol as opposed to abstaining is somewhat more acceptable now than when this book was first published, although in some circles it is still frowned on. I believe this is positive because giving people a choice in how they decide to help themselves makes addressing their drinking problem less scary and, as a result, increases the number of people who are willing to do something about it. Many people simply would not consider changing their use of alcohol if abstinence were the only way. I am not for or against abstinence, nor am I for or against moderation. I am for helping people figure out what they need to do, whether this involves learning to moderate their drinking or achieving abstinence. It is my hope that this new edition will fulfill my three reasons for writing the book originally by providing even more assistance to people who want to resolve their drinking problem.

HOW TO TELL IF YOU NEED THIS BOOK

According to the National Institute on Alcohol Abuse and Alcoholism, approximately 15.1 million adults in the United States have an alcohol use disorder. And for each of these individuals, there are many others who are at risk for severe consequences related to drinking. These are problem drinkers who don't quite meet the criteria for having an alcohol use disorder but who sometimes or frequently exceed moderate and safe drinking levels.

Many of these people know and admit that they have an alcohol problem, yet they simply do not want to see a therapist. Nor do they want to attend AA or other self-help meetings. Whether it is the stigma of having an alcohol problem, not knowing whom to turn to, wanting to do things themselves, or objecting to the cost of treatment, they do not get the help they need. If you are among the individuals in this group, this book is for you. It will help you to help yourself with your drinking in the privacy of your own home.

Other people are not sure whether they have a problem with alcohol consumption. While they have noticed patterns of drinking that worry them, they do not know whether alcohol is truly a problem for them. They are not ready or willing to enter the world of treatment or self-help. If you are among those individuals, this book also is for you. It will help you decide whether you have a drinking problem and, if you do, what you can do about it.

Perhaps you see yourself as having a drinking problem and have seen a therapist, but your treatment did not go well. Or perhaps you attended AA or other self-help meetings, but those did not go well either. You may feel discouraged and may have given up on yourself. Whatever problems you may have had with drinking and whatever treatment you may have had, this book is for you. It will help you answer the following questions.

Do You Have an Alcohol Problem?
Chapter 1 will help you make a realistic appraisal of whether you have a drinking problem and, if so, the extent of it. You will be asked to reflect in detail on your past drinking and any difficulties you have experienced that were in any way related to your use of alcohol. You will also begin to evaluate the damage your alcohol consumption

may have done to yourself and to your relationships. By the end of this chapter you will know whether your use of alcohol is problematic and whether you need to change your pattern of drinking.

If You Have an Alcohol Problem, Why Is This So?

Many individuals who have a problem with alcohol consumption wonder why they do. Chapter 2 reviews the prevailing ideas and explanations for some people's difficulty with controlling their alcohol intake. The goal is to help you understand why you may have a drinking problem and ensure that you do not beat yourself up for it. Chapter 3 expands on that discussion by reviewing the concept of self-medication, which is often used to explain why a person drinks too much.

Where to Begin?

Many people recognize that they have an alcohol problem but just don't know where to start. For example, they wonder how to get and stay motivated. In fact, having some mixed feelings about changing is common. A part of you wants to change, but another part of you wants to keep things the way they have always been. It is also easy for motivation to slacken after you get started. Chapter 4 helps you understand why this happens and how to stay on course.

People also often wonder whether it is possible to help themselves or whether they need to get treatment. The truth is that many people have been able to help themselves without outside assistance of any kind. Research has shown that about 75 percent of people with alcohol-related problems who recover do so without any formal help. In fact, not only is it possible for you to help yourself with your drinking problem, but truly you *must* help yourself. Whether you seek help from others or try to stop or moderate your drinking on your own, your success will rest primarily with you.

Chapter 5 explodes the myth that treatment is essential and cites studies showing that many people with drinking problems are able to help themselves. More important, it outlines the mental state that you will need to have if you are going to be successful. Chapter 6 helps you decide whether you will need medical assistance to stop your intake of alcohol safely. Whatever course you take, freeing yourself from the toxicity of alcohol will be crucial to your success.

Another question is whether completely stopping alcohol must be the way to go or whether you could try to moderate your drinking by learning to drink less. Chapter 7 considers this question and helps you decide how you should proceed.

Abstinence or Moderation?

This book offers specific plans to help you either moderate your drinking or stop drinking entirely. Because many people first want to try to moderate their drinking, or need to try it before considering abstinence, these strategies are presented first (chapters 8–10). If instead you decide that you would do better by learning how to abstain completely from alcohol, or if your attempt to moderate your drinking is not successful, turn to the techniques that will teach you how to stop drinking (chapters 11–14).

What If You Need Treatment or Want Outside Help?

For a number of reasons, some people want outside help or discover that, despite their best efforts, they need the assistance of others. In the next four chapters (15–18), I offer advice for those seeking treatment, and I review the variety of treatment options that are available to you to help you make the best choice. Being an informed consumer and being able to ask the right questions will help you get the help you need—if that is necessary.

What about Marijuana?

A question that often arises among people who have addressed their drinking is whether they can use another drug, specifically marijuana, without it affecting their recovery from their alcohol use disorder. With the legalization of marijuana in some states for medical or even recreational use, this question has come up more often.

While research on this issue is still at an early stage, in the final chapter, I review what is known and offer some tentative advice and recommendations.

A FINAL NOTE

This book is the result of many years of my experience successfully working with people who have suffered from their alcohol consumption. This book is also based on research into alcohol use and its treatment. It is true that some of what I say in this book is controversial. Not all professionals or paraprofessionals who work in the field agree with everything presented here. But my suggestions are not any less valid because of this, and they can help you if you heed them, work hard, and are honest with yourself. As you read this book, remember that your firm commitment to change is essential and that you must never lose sight of this.

Let your journey begin.

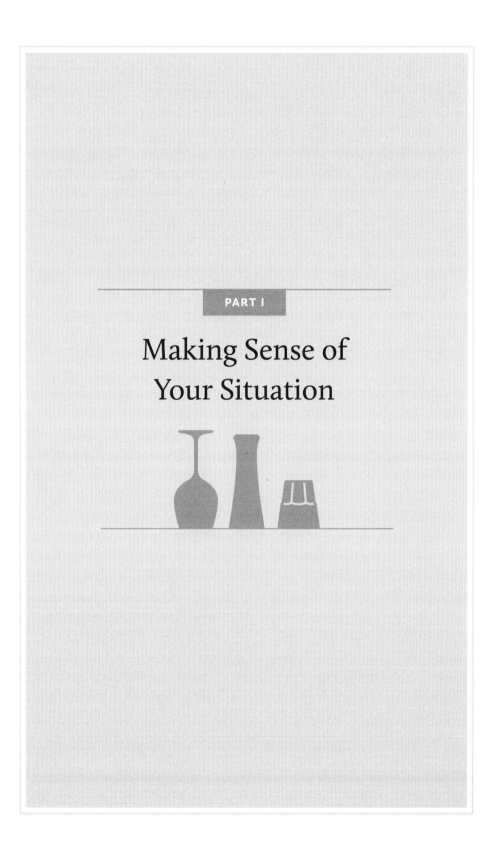

PART I

Making Sense of
Your Situation

Do You Have a Drinking Problem?

You can never learn less, you can only learn more.
R. Buckminster Fuller

Making the commitment to look at yourself and your relationship to alcohol is difficult. No one wants to admit that their drinking might be a problem. In some sectors of society, there is a stigma attached to having an alcohol problem, and you may feel that there is something wrong with you because you cannot always control your drinking. Drinking also probably plays an important role in your lifestyle, and most of your social activities may revolve around drinking. In fact, most of the friends you have may like to drink, and drinking is probably an important activity when you see them. There is a part of you that loves to drink, whether it is the taste, the excitement, the feeling you get from alcohol, the social lubricant it provides, the relaxation, the pain it masks, or some other desire that drinking fulfills. The reason you are thinking about your drinking comes not from your sudden dislike for alcohol. It is because your drinking is causing you problems.

This is an important distinction that I review in more detail in chapter 3. For now, keep in mind that your decision to look more closely at your drinking probably has little if anything to do with your wish to drink. You love to drink, and in the best of all worlds, you would continue to drink as you always have. If your drinking caused no problems, you would not even consider changing how you drink.

Eliminating the problems that arise from your drinking is the reason you have arrived at this crossroads.

People who go on diets do not choose to eat less or to eat different kinds of food because they no longer like to eat. They would love to continue to eat the way they always have. Rather, they choose to eat differently because they are sick and tired of being overweight. It is the consequences of eating too much that make them decide to eat differently.

Or take the person with a gambling problem who makes the decision to stop gambling. This person doesn't decide to do this because gambling is no longer fun and exciting. People who gamble too much are those who love to gamble. But they make the decision to stop gambling because it is causing significant destruction to their lives.

Obviously, you need to decide whether you even have a drinking problem. There is a fine line between a heavy social drinker and a problem drinker. Two common views about what describes a person with an alcohol use problem are, first, the inability to predict what will happen when you drink and, second, continuing to drink despite its harmful consequences for you. As you read the rest of the chapter, think about your past drinking experiences and be totally honest with yourself. Consider whether any of the examples apply to you.

THE INABILITY TO PREDICT
WHAT WILL HAPPEN WHEN YOU DRINK

A person is said to have a drinking problem if that person cannot always and consistently predict how much he or she will drink and what will happen once drinking begins. Individuals who fit this description drink regularly and generally without difficulty, yet they sometimes or often

— stay out later than intended, and this causes an argument with a spouse, girlfriend, boyfriend, or another significant other;

—go to a bar with others to have just one or two drinks but
continue drinking for hours and become very drunk;

—become mean or obnoxious when they drink;

—go for months without drinking, but when they start to
drink again, it soon gets out of control once more;

—miss work, school, or another important commitment
because of hangovers;

—drink too much, which causes shame and embarrassment;

—regret something they did or said while intoxicated;

—feel so physically bad the day after drinking that the day is
wasted; or

—drink so much that they can't remember what happened or
how they got home.

It is not that you always drink too much but that you can't *consistently avoid* drinking too much. Often your drinking is under control and may not cause you any difficulties, but at other times you drink too much, and there is a pattern of experiencing problems because of your drinking. You just can't seem to maintain control of your drinking in ways that do not cause you problems.

Tom is a 34-year-old married man and the father of 1-year-old twins. He had been a heavy social drinker while he was single. He had spent most weekends, and occasional weekdays, at bars with his friends he'd known since high school. After getting married at age 29, he purposely decreased his drinking because his wife, Sally, wasn't into the bar scene. He was able to limit his drinking on most occasions, but occasionally when he went out without Sally, he found himself staying at the bar until late at night and getting intoxicated, even though he had told Sally that he would be home after only a couple of drinks. He was able to limit his overdrinking episodes to about once per month, but this pattern was beginning to affect his marriage. And despite his repeated attempts not to let this happen, it still did—over and over again. Tom just couldn't *consistently* and *reliably* control his drinking.

Another example is Kim, a 37-year-old woman who has been married to Jeff for eight years. Over the years, Kim and Jeff seemed to drift away from each other, at least in part because they didn't openly communicate with each other about some issues that were going on in their relationship. Kim generally would get home from work well before Jeff, who would often meet some friends after work and not get home until much later. Whether due to Jeff's late arrivals or not, Kim got into a pattern of drinking wine when making dinner. While on most occasions Kim controlled her alcohol intake, several times each month she drank too much and was quite intoxicated when Jeff got home. Not only did this cause tension in the relationship, but when Kim was intoxicated, she would also express her anger, which caused even more difficulties. And in spite of numerous promises and attempts not to overdrink, Kim still did, which resulted in even more tension and conflict.

A final example is Dave, a 34-year-old man who has been married to Lori for six years with their two young children, ages 2 and 4. Due to intermittent heavy and problematic drinking, when he had engaged in reckless behavior such as driving when intoxicated and then feeling miserable after three days of drinking, he would often go for periods of not drinking that lasted from two to six months. After being "good" for these periods of time, he would come to believe that he could drink again without losing control. He would limit his drinking to the weekends and to having just a few drinks, but inevitably, after several weeks, his drinking would get completely out of control again.

It's Time to Be Honest with Yourself

Think about yourself and be completely honest. Do any of the examples listed on pages 16–17 or do the cases of Tom, Kim, or Dave describe your responses to alcohol? However hard you have tried to avoid problems as a result of drinking, have serious problems arisen anyway? If you answer yes, then you clearly need to address your drinking. This is true regardless of excuses such as "I hadn't eaten anything all day" or "I don't drink that much most of the time" or "I hadn't been out in months."

HARMFUL CONSEQUENCES RELATED TO DRINKING

People who continue to consume alcohol in spite of the harmful consequences related to their drinking have a drinking problem. These consequences can affect their professional, social, legal, physical, or financial life. People who fall into this category continue to drink even though they

— spend so much money on alcohol that there is not enough money for other things;

— obtain information from a physician that their liver is in trouble because of consuming too much alcohol;

— argue or fight with a spouse, girlfriend, or boyfriend about their alcohol consumption;

— miss work or school after a night of alcohol consumption because they feel so miserable;

— experience shakes or tremors caused by alcohol withdrawal;

— lose a job because of their drinking;

— alienate friends and family with their drinking;

— get arrested or involved in legal difficulties because of alcohol; or

— do things under the influence of alcohol that they later regret.

Chantal, a woman I started counseling after she was arrested for drunk driving a second time, was a 24-year-old single woman who had first started drinking when she was 16. She told me that she'd always loved the taste of alcohol and the feeling it gave her. She had fun with it and was never concerned about her drinking. She drank three or four times each week with her friends. She never experienced any problems related to alcohol until she was in her early twenties, when she was arrested for drunk driving. Still, she didn't think alcohol was a problem and attributed her arrest to a case of bad luck and being in the wrong place at the wrong time.

Over the next several years, Chantal's drinking escalated, and she admitted to me that she had lost several boyfriends because of her drinking. When drunk, she became flirtatious. And when her boyfriends had confronted her about it, she got angry and defensive, which eventually ended those relationships. Her drinking had caused problems with some of her girlfriends as well. When intoxicated, Chantal's behavior and attitude changed, and she became argumentative and nasty. She eventually was arrested again for drunk driving, which finally led her to admit that she had a drinking problem.

Analyzing Your Relationship with Alcohol

Does Chantal's situation or do any of the statements listed on page 19 describe your experiences? The important point to remember in assessing a drinking problem is the *quality* of your drinking rather than the absolute *quantity* of alcohol you consume. The interaction between you and alcohol is what makes alcohol consumption a problem or not.

For example, if you drink only once or twice a year, but it causes problems, then drinking is a problem. On the other hand, if you drink almost daily, but your drinking has never caused you or anyone one else any concerns, then you may not have an alcohol problem.

The criteria for deciding whether you have a drinking problem are what happens when you drink and what problems alcohol causes for you. If you can be totally honest with yourself, it is not difficult to decide whether drinking is a problem for you.

TAKING THE TEST

The MAST
Questionnaires have been developed to help people assess whether alcohol use is a problem. One is the MAST, or the Michigan Alcoholism Screening Test (see pages 22–23). Take this test *now, before* reading the next two paragraphs, and answer the 25 questions honestly.

To score this test, give yourself two points for each "no" answer to questions 1, 4, 6, and 8. For the rest of the questions, give yourself two points for each question you answered "yes" to, except give yourself one point for questions 3, 5, 10, and 17 and five points for questions 9, 20, and 21. And don't score question 7 regardless of how you answer it; this question was found to be unhelpful in determining who had an alcohol problem or who did not. Based on their score, a person can be classified as not having a problem (0–3), maybe having a problem (3–4), or probably having a problem (5 and above).

How did you do? Based on your score, do you think that you might need to do something about your drinking? If you earned at least five points, your drinking is a problem.

The AUDIT
Another test for identifying individuals with an alcohol use disorder is the AUDIT, or the Alcohol Use Disorders Identification Test (see pages 24–25). Again, take the test now before reading how it is scored in the next two paragraphs. Answer the 10 questions as honestly as you can.

On this test, scores for questions 1–8 range from zero to four, with the first answer option for each question scoring zero, the second scoring one, the third scoring two, the fourth scoring three, and the last scoring four. For questions 9 and 10, which only have three answer options, the scoring is zero for the first option, two for the next one, and four for the last one.

A score of 8 or more is associated with harmful or hazardous drinking, with a score of 13 or more for women and a score of 15 or more for men indicating a more serious alcohol use disorder.

Michigan Alcoholism Screening Test

1. Do you feel you are a normal drinker?	Yes	No
2. Have you ever awakened in the morning after some drinking the night before and found that you could not remember part of the evening?	Yes	No
3. Does your wife/husband or parents ever worry or complain about your drinking?	Yes	No
4. Can you stop drinking without a struggle after one or two drinks?	Yes	No
5. Do you ever feel bad about your drinking?	Yes	No
6. Do your friends or relatives think that you are a normal drinker?	Yes	No
7. Do you ever try to limit your drinking to certain times of the day or to certain places?	Yes	No
8. Are you always able to stop when you want to?	Yes	No
9. Have you ever attended a meeting of Alcoholics Anonymous?	Yes	No
10. Have you gotten into fights when drinking?	Yes	No
11. Has drinking ever created problems with you and your wife/husband?	Yes	No
12. Has your wife/husband or other family members ever gone to anyone for help about your drinking?	Yes	No
13. Have you ever lost friends or girlfriends/boyfriends because of your drinking?	Yes	No
14. Have you ever gotten into trouble at work because of drinking?	Yes	No
15. Have you ever lost a job because of drinking?	Yes	No
16. Have you ever neglected your obligations, your family, or work for two days or more in a row because of drinking?	Yes	No
17. Do you ever drink before noon?	Yes	No

18. Have you ever been told you have liver trouble?   Yes   No

19. Have you ever had DTs (delirium tremens), severe shaking, heard voices, or seen things that weren't there after heavy drinking?   Yes   No

20. Have you ever gone to anyone for help about your drinking?   Yes   No

21. Have you ever been in a hospital because of drinking?   Yes   No

22. Have you ever been a patient in a psychiatric hospital or a psychiatric ward of a general hospital where drinking was part of the problem?   Yes   No

23. Have you ever been at a psychiatric or mental health clinic, or gone to a doctor or clergyman for help with an emotional problem in which drinking has played a part?   Yes   No

24. Have you ever been arrested, even for a few hours, because of drunken behavior?   Yes   No

25. Have you ever been arrested for drunken driving or driving after drinking?   Yes   No

Alcohol Use Disorders Identification Test

Please mark the answer that is correct for you

1. How often do you have a drink containing alcohol?
   ☐ Never
   ☐ Monthly or less
   ☐ 2–4 times a month
   ☐ 2–3 times a week
   ☐ 4 or more times a week

2. How many standard drinks containing alcohol do you have on a typical day when drinking?
   ☐ 1 or 2
   ☐ 3 or 4
   ☐ 5 or 6
   ☐ 7 to 9
   ☐ 10 or more

3. How often do you have six or more drinks on one occasion?
   ☐ Never
   ☐ Less than monthly
   ☐ Monthly
   ☐ Weekly
   ☐ Daily or almost daily

4. During the past year, how often have you found that you were not able to stop drinking once you had started?
   ☐ Never
   ☐ Less than monthly
   ☐ Monthly
   ☐ Weekly
   ☐ Daily or almost daily

5. During the past year, how often have you failed to do what was normally expected of you because of drinking?
   ☐ Never
   ☐ Less than monthly
   ☐ Monthly
   ☐ Weekly
   ☐ Daily or almost daily

6. During the past year, how often have you needed a drink in the morning to get yourself going after a heavy drinking session?
   □ Never
   □ Less than monthly
   □ Monthly
   □ Weekly
   □ Daily or almost daily

7. During the past year, how often have you had a feeling of guilt or remorse after drinking?
   □ Never
   □ Less than monthly
   □ Monthly
   □ Weekly
   □ Daily or almost daily

8. During the past year, have you been unable to remember what happened the night before because you had been drinking?
   □ Never
   □ Less than monthly
   □ Monthly
   □ Weekly
   □ Daily or almost daily

9. Have you or someone else been injured as a result of your drinking?
   □ No
   □ Yes, but not in the past year
   □ Yes, during the past year

10. Has a relative or friend, doctor or other health worker been concerned about your drinking or suggested you cut down?
    □ No
    □ Yes, but not in the past year
    □ Yes, during the past year

From AUDIT, available at https://auditscreen.org/about/faqs/.

How did you do? Does your score suggest that you have a drinking problem and that it is time to do something about it?

The CAGE
Another simple screening test is called the CAGE, which you can take now.

CAGE

Have you ever felt that you should **C**ut down on your drinking?

Have people **A**nnoyed you by criticizing your drinking?

Have you ever felt bad or **G**uilty about your drinking?

Have you ever had a drink first thing in the morning to "steady your nerves" or get rid of a hangover (**E**yeopener)?

Used with permission from Ewing, J. A. (1984). Detecting alcoholism. The CAGE questionnaire. *Journal of the American Medical Association, 252*(14): 1905–1907.

So, how did you do on the CAGE? Did you answer yes to any of the questions? If you did, your drinking is causing you problems.

Even though questionnaires of this kind can be helpful, they are not as important as you truthfully looking at yourself. You don't need a questionnaire to know if you are overweight, if you are happy with your job, or if you are satisfied with your financial situation. Likewise, you won't need a questionnaire to determine whether drinking is a problem for you when you have the courage to be honest with yourself.

BUT I'M NOT THAT BAD!

Maybe you found when you took these tests and honestly looked at yourself that your drinking does affect you and others but that you still function pretty well. You discovered that while alcohol does cause you some problems, you aren't that bad. You still work every day, meet your financial obligations, and are generally successful. In fact, you know others who have a much more serious alcohol problem than you have. Nonetheless you need to know that

- most people who struggle with the consequences of drinking continue to work and meet their financial obligations;

- they do not drink every day and, in many ways, continue to fulfill most of their responsibilities;

- they are often successful in many realms of their life; and

- the image of the skid-row drunk fits only a small percentage of people who have a serious alcohol problem.

Remember: Although alcohol may not affect every aspect of your life, it can still clearly cause damage to your life. Don't allow the thought "I am not that bad" prevent you from doing something about your drinking.

SUMMARY

If you cannot always predict how much you will drink or what will happen when you do, or if your drinking causes serious difficulties for you and others around you, you have an alcohol use problem. It is just that simple. If you have any doubts, reread this chapter and answer the three questionnaires again and see how you score. And remember that you do not need to experience all of these difficulties to conclude that you have a drinking problem. Even occasional problems, when they happen over and over again, qualify.

It is time for you to be completely honest with yourself. Only your truthful evaluation of past drinking and its effect on your life can lead you forward. If you are candid with yourself, you will have no difficulty deciding whether your alcohol consumption is something you need to address, either by learning to drink moderately or by abstaining from alcohol.

If you conclude that you have a problem with alcohol, you may wonder, "Why does drinking cause *me* problems, while others seem to be able to drink moderately and without any difficulty?" "Why am I different?" "Why do I drink too much?" "Why can't I drink like others do?" Or "what is wrong with me?"

There are two perspectives on problematic drinking that help you answer these questions: the disease perspective and the learned behavior perspective. There is also one other perspective that you should not consider: the personal weakness perspective. The next chapter helps you understand yourself, and that understanding will determine how you can deal with your drinking problem, now that you know you have one.

CHAPTER 2

Why Does Drinking Cause You Difficulty?

There are no eternal facts as there are no absolute truths.
FRIEDRICH NIETZSCHE

Okay. So you have honestly looked at yourself and realized that your drinking is hurting you. Maybe you don't always run into trouble when you drink, but this often happens, and you have noticed a destructive pattern. The next question is "Why?" Why can't you consistently control your consumption of alcohol? What is wrong with you? Why can't you drink like others who don't experience problems when they drink?

Some people may wonder whether they are an *alcoholic*, whatever that word really means. So often, after it becomes clear that a person I see in therapy has a problem with alcohol, that person either wants to know if they are an alcoholic or they say something like this to me: "I know I have a problem with drinking, but I am not an *alcoholic*," as though it is a dirty word. I have witnessed heated discussions between spouses, where a wife, for example, accuses her husband of being an alcoholic, and the husband vehemently denies it. I have also met people who find that acknowledging they are alcoholics provides them with relief and comfort.

In this chapter, to help you make sense of your situation, I review the two main perspectives on why some people have a problem with alcohol. This understanding will help you develop a course of action. Before I do this, though, I want first to describe a point of view that is prevalent in society but that is not true and that you should not

29

hold. This perspective is destructive, and if you already believe it, you should dispel it from your mind.

THE PERSONAL WEAKNESS PERSPECTIVE

A common belief is that people who drink too much are abnormal. Unlike "normal" healthy people who drink without difficulty, people who overdrink do not control their alcohol use and allow it to get the best of them. The inability to control alcohol intake is believed to stem from some kind of personal weakness. This idea may not be verbalized, but the belief exists nevertheless: there must be something wrong with people who drink too much, and if they can figure out what is wrong, they will be able to stop their destructive drinking.

This perspective focuses on personal *choice*. People, the belief goes, "choose" whether to drink too much. And if they choose to drink too much and cause problems for themselves, others, and society, then they are irresponsible and lacking in some way. It follows that they must be weak people because they do not control their use of alcohol. The social stigma attached to having an alcohol abuse problem originates from this belief.

An Illogical Idea

Although the personal weakness perspective is popular in many segments of our society, there is a huge logical problem with this point of view: *many, many people who have a drinking problem show incredible strength and fortitude in other areas of their life.* For example, many successful businesspeople, professional athletes, physicians, and entertainers have or have had a drinking problem. These people have demonstrated a powerful will to succeed and have shown personal determination in many aspects of their life. They have accomplished much, and sometimes, even despite drinking, they continue to achieve and appear successful. It is hard to make sense of this if all individuals who have a drinking problem are weak people.

Also, lots of people who have messed up their life with alcohol one day resolve their drinking problem and begin to flourish and blossom. They achieve what they want to and become successful. If they were truly weak people, this simply wouldn't be possible.

Human Nature

It is human nature for people to struggle with an inability to control their behavior at some time in their lives. For example, common problems include being unable to control aggression, feeling anxious about speaking in front of an audience, being afraid to speak one's mind in a conflict situation, overworking, or compulsively exercising, to name just a few. If we do not consider these people weak or lacking in character strength, then you should not consider yourself weak or lacking in character strength just because you have a drinking problem.

Nearly everyone can get stuck in a certain way of being in the world. Sigmund Freud, the father of psychoanalysis, noted this more than a century ago. He found that people often repeat the same behavior over and over despite suffering from its adverse consequences. Freud named this the "repetition compulsion." Struggling with an alcohol problem is one way of being stuck, not necessarily a sign of being weak or defective in some way.

A Vulnerability to Addiction

There is a vulnerability to addiction in our species, and people who struggle with addiction are not weak people. Rather, getting addicted to things defines who we are. When you look at the causes of *preventable* death in the United States, the top three behaviors that lead to preventable death are

- Smoking tobacco

- Poor diet and physical inactivity leading to obesity

- Excessive alcohol use

Smoking, poor eating habits, and excessive alcohol use can all be addictions, and if this doesn't suggest that humans have a propensity to get addicted to things, I don't know what does. Despite the severe ramifications of continuing to engage in these behaviors, many people struggle to change their behavior. The list of potential addictions also includes shopping, gambling, surfing the internet, pornography, drinking coffee, and even work. Sometimes a healthy activity like exercise can become an addiction if a person continues to exercise despite a warning from a doctor to take some time off after an injury.

Are all people who struggle with an addiction weak? That is, is the individual who continues to smoke tobacco weak? Or how about the person who struggles with weight control? If these people are not viewed as weak, then the person who struggles with alcohol should not be viewed that way either.

The point is that many people struggle with some kind of addiction. Viewing these people as weak or lacking in some way makes no sense, and similarly, you should not view yourself in such a way.

A Dangerous Trap

Don't buy into the personal weakness point of view. The worst thing you can do is "beat yourself up" for drinking too much or believe that you are a weak person because you drink too much. This will only make you feel worse about who you are and will damage your sense of self. In fact, you may even fall into the trap of drinking more to cope with feeling so bad. This is why the personal weakness perspective is so destructive.

Rather than viewing yourself as weak, it is important that you see yourself as having a drinking problem caused by a variety of complex factors that you do not fully understand. Consider your drinking to be your way of coping with forces just beyond your grasp. You are no different from people who struggle with other problems in life. Perhaps you need to develop new coping skills and ideas about yourself, which may include viewing your problem with alcohol a little differently.

THE DISEASE PERSPECTIVE

The most widely held understanding about an alcohol problem throughout Western culture is that it is a disease. The name given to this disease is *alcoholism*. The idea that a drinking problem is a disease is held by the American Medical Association, American Psychiatric Association, American Public Health Association, American Hospital Association, American Psychological Association, National Association of Social Workers, World Health Organization, American College of Physicians, and American Society of Addiction Medicine.

So what does it mean to say that a drinking problem is a disease? According to *Webster's Dictionary*, a disease is a condition of the body or one of its parts that impairs the performance of a vital function. Clearly, while under the influence of alcohol, the brain is not functioning well. Also, over time, alcohol can damage most every organ in your body. Calling a drinking problem a disease does not, however, describe what the disease is all about or what causes it.

You're Born with It

For many, the disease of alcoholism is an inherited biological vulnerability that predisposes a person to developing a problem with alcohol. This biological vulnerability interacts with a person's living situation, culture, and emotions and causes the person to drink too much. From this perspective, it is not the alcoholic's fault that he or she cannot drink responsibly and with control. Such individuals have an illness that makes them unable to handle their liquor and drink in moderation. Although the mechanism by which this happens is not completely understood, for these individuals, even one drink may lead to a loss of control over their drinking. That is, one drink will lead to more drinking, and eventually the use of alcohol becomes uncontrolled and takes over the person.

For Many, the Disease Is Chronic, Progressive, and Fatal

- Chronic: It is always there. You have it for life, and it doesn't go away.

- Progressive: It will get worse and worse over time if left untreated.

- Fatal: You can die from it if it is left untreated.

F. Scott Fitzgerald wrote, "First you take a drink, then the drink takes a drink, then the drink takes you." In other words, drinking can take over your life, and eventually, it can kill you.

For Others, the Disease Is There, but . . .
While many people have a severe form of the disease that is chronic, progressive, and fatal, for others, the disease may have a less cruel course. While the use of alcohol will continue to complicate their life, it may not get worse and worse and lead to death. Like most any illness, symptoms can vary along a continuum, from mild, to moderate, to severe. For example, asthma, cancer, diabetes, obesity, and high cholesterol affect people, but the severity of these disorders and their impact on a person can vary. Some have a very dangerous and precarious form of the illness, whereas for others, the overall harshness of the disorder is less extreme.

In fact, an alcohol use disorder used to be conceived as either "alcohol abuse" or "alcohol dependence." However, it is now understood as falling somewhere on a spectrum. The point is that from the disease perspective, you can have the disease because of an inherited biological vulnerability, but it can vary in terms of severity.

Alcoholism through the Ages
The idea that excessive drinking may be a disease was first noted more than 200 years ago.

- From the late 1700s to the early 1800s, Dr. Benjamin Rush, whom the temperance movement (1845–1918) claimed as its founder, was among the first to write about it. He wrote that while drinking was first the effect of "free agency," eventually the habit turned into a necessity and was a "disease of the will." He also prescribed abstinence as the only cure.

- In 1838, Samuel B. Woodward, superintendent of a mental asylum in Worcester, Massachusetts, and perhaps the leading mental health physician of the time, wrote a series of articles that described alcohol addiction as a "physical disease." He also wrote that the desire for alcohol could be so uncontrollable that it was questionable whether the power of the will could fight the desire to drink.

- In the early 1900s, the idea that alcoholism was a disease continued to be accepted within the psychiatric and social work fields, although the specifics of it had not been fully worked out. It is fair to say, though, that the cause of alcoholism was believed to be alcohol, owing to its power to take over someone's will.

- In the 1930s and 1940s, ideas about the cause of alcoholism began to shift. With a renewed interest in alcohol problems in the United States, in large part due to the development of AA and the Yale Center of Alcohol Studies, researchers started to revise their understanding and began to believe that the disease of alcoholism was something that occurred only to some people for unclear reasons.

- In 1960, E. M. Jellinek, the founder of the Center of Alcohol Studies and Summer School of Alcohol Studies, originally at Yale and by then at Rutgers University, published his book, *The Disease Concept of Alcoholism*, which outlined the medical model of alcoholism. He identified several different types of alcoholics. According to him, some individuals experienced a "loss of control," in which any drinking began a chain reaction that led to more and more drinking, which made it impossible to control alcohol intake. He also noted that the cause of some types of alcoholism may be inherited.

- In 1976, the American Society of Addiction Medicine (ASAM), the leading group of physicians in the United States dedicated to the understanding and treatment of substance use problems, developed a definition of alcoholism that called it a disease.

- In 1990, the ASAM modified its definition of alcoholism to state that heredity was involved and that alcoholism was an involuntary disability marked by an inability to control drinking consistently.

Is a Drinking Problem an Inherited Condition?

Is it possible that your heredity could be responsible for your overdrinking? And if this is true, how does your genetic makeup play a role? These are complicated questions, and there is still much that we have to learn. But let me tell you what is currently known.

First, it is clear that heredity is important. We know that children of alcoholic parents who are adopted at birth and raised by nonalcoholic parents have a much greater probability of developing alcoholism than do children of nonalcoholic parents who are adopted at birth and raised by alcoholic parents. So heredity is important, even more than the environment in which one grows up.

One study followed a group of adolescent boys for about 40 years. The adolescents were given a variety of psychological tests, and their families were also assessed. As these individuals matured, some developed serious problems with alcohol, and others did not. It was found that the rate of serious alcohol problems among men who had two or more alcohol-abusing relatives was about three times higher than among men who had no alcohol-abusing relatives. In fact, one of the best predictors of developing a problem with alcohol is coming from a family in which one or more members have had a problem with alcohol. In most cases, people I have seen who struggle with alcohol report that biological relatives have had drinking problems.

Studies of twins have also shown that genes are important by comparing the rates of alcohol problems among identical twins with the rates of alcohol problems among fraternal twins. Identical twins share the same genes, but fraternal twins do not. Therefore, if alcohol problems are largely biologically determined, both members of a set of identical twins will more often have alcohol problems than will both members of a set of fraternal twins.

Again, the results were clear: there is a higher rate of shared alcohol problems for identical twins when one of them has a problem than for fraternal twins when one has a problem, which supports the idea that alcohol problems are at least in part biologically and genetically determined.

An Alcohol Problem Is Not Unlike Other Medical Illnesses

Research has demonstrated that heredity is an important factor for many illnesses. In addition, it has been found that the genetic contribution to the risk of developing an alcohol problem is similar to the genetic contribution to the risk of developing hypertension, asthma, and diabetes.

For example, research has shown that 25–50 percent of the risk for developing hypertension comes from one's genetic makeup. For type 1 diabetes, heritability estimates range 30–55 percent, and for type 2 diabetes, the estimate is 80 percent. Heritability estimates for developing adult-onset asthma are 36–70 percent. When examining the impact of genes on developing an alcohol problem among men, research has shown that about 55 percent of the risk is due to heredity. Thus, it is clear that many illnesses have important genetic determinants, and the genetic risk of developing an alcohol problem is similar to the risk for a number of other illnesses.

How Does Heredity Increase the Risk of Developing an Alcohol Problem?

So if heredity is partly responsible for someone developing a problem with alcohol, how does this work? What is inherited that causes a person to overdrink?

Often the children of parents who have alcohol problems, who presumably have a biological vulnerability to overdrinking, feel less intoxicated when they drink the same amount of alcohol as people with no family history of drinking problems. Alcohol simply affects them less, and they can drink a lot without feeling particularly intoxicated. It follows that this ability to handle alcohol, which is biologically based and inherited, may lead them to drink more than others to obtain the same effect from alcohol. This leads to increased rates of drinking and drinking problems.

The "Hollow Leg" Syndrome

You may have heard of the "hollow leg" syndrome, in which some people seem to be able to put away huge quantities of alcohol in their so-called hollow leg without showing signs of gross intoxication. You yourself may be able to drink a lot more than others you know who get drunk after only a few drinks. While some consider this ability a source of pride and a sign of personal strength, in truth, it is a sign of a potential drinking problem.

People with different responses to alcohol have been studied over many years to see whether those who can drink a lot without feeling intoxicated have a greater chance of developing alcohol problems. Once again, the evidence is clear: people who have a low response to alcohol have a much greater chance of becoming alcoholic compared with people who get intoxicated after only one or two drinks.

Even though people with a low response to alcohol can drink more than others, the amount of alcohol they consume often catches up to them eventually. What I mean is that while *initially* the person does not feel intoxicated *even after having many drinks*, in due course and often quite suddenly, the person can get grossly intoxicated, experience a blackout, and encounter problems.

I am reminded of Justin, a young man who was referred to me after having experienced an incident at college. Justin was 21 years old and in his last year of college. While he could not remember everything that happened, he had been charged with breaking some windows of his dorm, was found passed out by a security guard, and was taken to the hospital. He was told to get a mental health evaluation as a condition of being allowed to return to school.

When I saw Justin and we reviewed his alcohol history, he reported that he could drink a lot more than his peers and that he tended to handle his alcohol intake rather well. He generally had not run into any trouble but did describe a few instances when he overdrank and experienced a blackout, not remembering the next day what had happened the evening before. He told me that he was a little concerned about this. He described one evening when he could not remember where he had parked his car or how he got back to college. He also mentioned to me that his father used to have a drinking problem but was currently abstinent from alcohol.

I talked with Justin about what a low response to alcohol was and asked him if he could drink a lot without feeling intoxicated and then, sometimes, have the effect hit him all at once. This idea immediately resonated with him, and his eyes lit up. He said this response described him exactly, and he realized that he must no longer drink or, if he did, be careful about the amount of alcohol he consumed.

Heredity May Also Be Responsible for How Much You Like Alcohol

When I work with people who struggle with alcohol, I am always interested in what they like about alcohol and how it makes them feel. This can often be a window into what they will need to experience in their life once alcohol is removed. For example, if a person says that alcohol is relaxing, this tells me the person may need to find other ways to unwind. Or if someone says that alcohol takes away feelings of stress associated with a particular issue in life, it is clear to me that the individual needs to address that issue in a healthier way.

While there are times when this line of questioning can be helpful, at other times people struggle to find words that explain what they like about drinking. I often hear people say that they just like the way alcohol makes them feel, the "buzz" it gives them, or they tell me that they simply don't know why. Alcohol grabs them and they like the feeling, but they can't put words to it. I have also heard from people who do not overdrink that they do not like how alcohol makes them feel. They may enjoy one drink, but they do not like the feeling of intoxication.

I have come to believe, a belief supported by research, that genetics may be largely responsible for how a person responds to the effects of alcohol. For some, alcohol has an amazing capacity to make them feel good. It can also take away their negative feelings. For others, however, alcohol simply does not have those kinds of pleasant effects.

The same is true with other substances that can be used to excess. Some people love the way that cocaine, for example, makes them feel, whereas others cannot tolerate it. There are individuals who take an opioid drug and have a feeling of euphoria. On the other hand, other people take the same drug and do not like the experience at all. I believe that neurochemistry, which is largely inherited, determines why, for some, alcohol is highly rewarding, and this obviously increases their risk of developing a drinking problem.

Nothing Happens in a Vacuum

We should also remember that the genetic susceptibility passed from parent to child must interact with psychological, social, and cultural factors in order to result in an alcohol problem. For example, you might have a predisposition to developing a drinking problem, but if you live in a society where drinking is frowned on or where alcohol simply is not available, you probably will never develop a drinking problem because you choose not to drink or cannot choose to drink. On the other hand, if you are biologically vulnerable and live in an environment where heavy drinking is common, you are far more likely to develop a problem with alcohol.

It is also possible that you may have experienced some distress in your life and found that drinking helped in some way and made you feel better. Or perhaps you experienced some physical pain and discovered that alcohol took the edge off and relieved your discomfort. Your biological vulnerability may have been awakened by these other factors and led to an alcohol problem. In fact, without these other variables, your alcohol problem may never have developed.

So, the reasons why someone develops an alcohol problem can be complicated. But regardless of the causes, the drinking-as-a-disease perspective places a heavy emphasis on heredity to explain why some people cannot consistently control their drinking.

So What Does This Mean for You?

It Isn't Your Fault. The drinking-as-a-disease perspective doesn't blame you or anyone for having an alcohol problem. It is not your fault that you cannot control your drinking because how your body reacts to alcohol is largely genetically determined. This perspective also emphasizes the importance of having compassion for the problem drinker rather than disdain. If we know anything, it is that support and compassion help people who drink too much.

It also means that you and others should not necessarily try to understand the root psychological causes of why you drink too much. Your problem is largely based on your heredity and biological tendency to drink excessively and crave alcohol.

Drinking Can't Be Controlled. If someone has the disease of alcoholism, drinking can't consistently be controlled. This loss of control is inevitable and largely defines the nature of the beast. No matter how hard you try, you have an inborn propensity to drink too much, and it will always be a challenge to control your drinking. So, the only way to avoid the problem is by never taking that first drink.

There Is No Going Back. If a person has the disease of alcoholism, there is no going back. There is an expression that once a cucumber changes into a pickle, the pickle can never go back to being a cucumber. Well, the same is true about alcoholism. Once a person becomes an alcoholic, that person can't ever go back to being a social drinker. Once this line is crossed, people must accept their condition and learn that they cannot drink safely.

No matter how hard you have tried to control your drinking, have you eventually returned to your old habits and problems? Do you think that you have the disease of alcoholism? If you do, abstinence is the only way to overcome your illness. There is no alternative, and this is your only solution.

THE LEARNED BEHAVIOR PERSPECTIVE

Human beings are creatures of learning. We learn how to walk, how to read, how to write, how to golf, how to swim, and how to play tennis. We also learn how to avoid pain, how to obtain pleasure, what makes us happy, and what makes us sad. We learn what kinds of food we like and what kinds of food we dislike. We learn the type of people we like to be with and, as important, the type of people we don't want to be around. And we even learn how to drink alcohol.

When I talk with people who struggle with drinking, I am always interested in how they discovered alcohol, what they like about drinking, and what influences played a role in how they learned to drink. Did they grow up in a household where alcohol flowed freely? Were many, if not most, of their peers into heavy drinking? Was drinking to get drunk the norm in their surroundings? Was it common to unwind after work by drinking? In some cultures, drunkenness is tolerated, if not encouraged, but in other societies, heavy drinking is discouraged. All of these influences play a role in how people learn to use alcohol.

Over the course of life, people learn how alcohol makes them feel, and some learn to use alcohol to enhance or take away certain feelings. For example, some people use alcohol as a way to decrease tension and stress. Others use it as a social lubricant that helps them feel more relaxed around others. Some may have discovered that alcohol helps them feel less depressed or gives them energy. And some people have learned that alcohol takes away their boredom and loneliness.

The learned behavior perspective maintains that, to a large degree, excessive drinking is unhealthy learned behavior. While this perspective may accept that some people have a greater chance of developing a problem with alcohol than others owing to their heredity, this perspective still views a drinking problem as largely learned.

Learned Behavior or a Disease—Who Cares?

So what does it matter if a drinking problem is learned behavior as opposed to a disease? It is important because the perspective that a drinking problem is learned behavior allows for the possibility that a person with a drinking problem may be able to learn to drink differently and drink less. If problematic drinking is learned, then some people may learn how to moderate their drinking. This contrasts with the drinking-as-a-disease perspective, which maintains that it is simply not possible for an alcoholic to drink differently. The only way to resolve a drinking problem from the disease perspective is by permanent abstinence from alcohol.

So Can a Pickle Be Turned Back into a Cucumber?

Although the drinking-as-a-disease perspective says it isn't possible, some people who have experienced a drinking problem have been able to change their pattern of alcohol use and have learned to drink differently. When people change their pattern of drinking, this change can take any number of forms, including

— drinking only occasionally, such as only on holidays or at special events;

— abstaining from alcohol for a period of time but eventually starting again with limited drinking;

— limiting drinking to weekends and having only a few drinks;

— drinking only in social settings where they know they won't overdo it;

— drinking several times per week but limiting the amount they drink; or

— changing the type of alcohol they drink.

Less important than how they are doing it is the fact that they are *able* to do this, which suggests that a drinking problem may be largely learned and that people can learn to drink differently and without problems.

What the Research Shows

Perhaps one of most famous studies showing that some problem drinkers could learn to drink differently was a study known as the RAND Report. The study examined more than 900 men who struggled with drinking and who had been treated in 45 alcohol treatment programs across the United States. These treatment programs all maintained that abstinence was the only way to resolve a drinking problem. Despite this treatment orientation, one-and-a-half years later a significant number of these men were drinking moderately, at amounts that were not destructive or out of control.

Another and even larger study looked at more than 2,000 individuals who had an alcohol problem but were no longer experiencing problems related to their drinking for at least one year. This sample was broken down into three groups: individuals who were abstinent; individuals who were drinking within the guidelines recommended by the National Institute on Alcohol and Alcoholism that define low-risk drinking (low-risk drinkers); and individuals who exceeded these guidelines (risky drinkers) but were not experiencing signs of problematic drinking. These same individuals were re-interviewed three years later to assess the status of their drinking.

About one-half of the low-risk drinkers had continued to drink in low-risk ways, and about half of the risky drinkers had either continued to drink that way or had decreased their drinking. Some had relapsed and others had decided to choose abstinence, but what is clear is that many continued to drink without harm despite having experienced an alcohol problem.

While three years is not that long, both studies were large and well designed, and they challenged the conventional wisdom maintaining that people who struggled with drinking would *immediately* resume out-of-control drinking after taking that first drink. Other, smaller studies have followed people with significant alcohol problems for many years and have found the same thing—that some people with a drinking problem are able to learn how to control their drinking. Perhaps some pickles can be turned back into cucumbers.

Can Old Dogs Be Taught New Tricks?
The RAND Report and other studies showed that old dogs can, by themselves, learn new tricks. Although their treatment had pushed abstinence, many study participants had instead learned how to control their drinking. But can people who struggle with alcohol be *taught* to drink less? The drinking-as-learned-behavior perspective holds that if drinking is learned, then treatment that tries to teach people how to drink less could possibly succeed. And, in fact, many people who have suffered from drinking too much have been taught to drink less with treatment that uses principles of learning.

What Does This Mean for You?
The drinking-as-learned-behavior perspective suggests that not all people who have an alcohol problem have the disease of alcoholism and therefore must abstain from alcohol to stop it from ruining their lives. This perspective questions the whole concept that a drinking problem is a disease. While heredity is relevant, this perspective views an alcohol problem as maladaptive behavior learned from a variety of sources: psychological, social, cultural, and educational. While abstinence may be the best policy for many, this perspective makes a place for the individual who can successfully learn how to drink moderately.

SO WHAT IS THE TRUTH?

So what is the truth? Should you view your drinking problem as a disease or as an unhealthy learned habit? This is a complicated question that only you can answer.

There Are Many Truths

I believe that the cause of an alcohol problem is complex and that there are different truths for different people. An alcohol problem can be caused by genetic, biological, psychological, or cultural factors, to name just a few, or by a combination of all of these. It is shortsighted and narrow-minded to think that there is only one way to understand a person's problem with alcohol. I also believe that whatever is passed on in the genes that makes someone susceptible to developing a problem with alcohol is multifaceted and varies along a continuum. For some, the genetic loading is extremely powerful; for others, it may take a milder form, although it still puts the person at a higher than average risk.

Find Your Own Truth

How you understand your problem with alcohol is a decision that only you can make, and your belief must benefit you and no one else. If you believe that your drinking problem is the result of a disease, then view it this way. For many individuals, the idea that they have a disease works because it provides a clear road to recovery. Because having a disease implies that you are not at fault, you may overcome any guilt (which you should not have anyway) as well.

I have seen many people with a destructive pattern of drinking who began drinking problematically at an early age, and they reported that drinking problems ran heavily in their family. They had repeatedly tried to moderate their drinking without success and could offer no explanation for why they could not control it, other than to say, "I am an alcoholic." The idea of having a disease was the only way they could understand themselves, and it fit for them.

I am reminded of Mitchell, who told me that from the time he first tasted alcohol he was a "blackout" drinker. He would drink to get drunk, and he would often experience blackouts in which he couldn't remember what he had done the night before or how he got home. As an adult, he would binge drink until he was so physically ill that he couldn't drink anymore. The only way Mitchell could understand himself was that he had the disease of alcoholism. He knew that if he continued to drink, he would eventually die from it.

You, on the other hand, may want to view your drinking as a bad habit you have learned, whether the reasons for it are psychological, cultural, or social. The idea of being diseased or alcoholic may not sit well with you. Having a disease may make you feel defective or abnormal. You may think that you could learn to control your drinking, and you may want to try.

However, even if you don't accept the idea that you have a disease, you can still choose abstinence to solve your problem. I have worked with people who could never "buy" the disease perspective yet who still chose to abstain from alcohol as the way to recover from their drinking problem. I am reminded of Sam, age 45, a successful individual who drank heavily and almost daily in his youth. Over time, he had limited his drinking to a few times a year. Still, every time he drank, he experienced difficulties. He finally chose abstinence as the way to recover from his problem, but he always understood his problem as a bad habit rather than a disease.

SUMMARY

In this chapter, I have tried to give you an understanding of why you have developed a problem with alcohol. The two main viewpoints for understanding why a person develops a drinking problem are the disease concept and the learned behavior perspective. The disease concept maintains that a drinking problem is largely an inherited condition, whereas the learned behavior perspective suggests that a drinking problem is a learned behavior, although genetics may still play a role. I have also described the personal weakness perspective, which I hope you now see is irrational. Believing that will only make you feel worse about yourself.

How you perceive your drinking problem must fit with your view of the world. How you choose to view your alcohol problem must help you and no one else. There aren't any right or wrong answers, unless your answers lead to more drinking problems.

In fact, although you may find it frustrating, you may never fully know why you have developed an alcohol problem, just like a tobacco smoker or someone who overeats may never fully understand why they have a problem either. And that is OK.

The most significant issue is not what you call your drinking problem, how you see it, or having a full understanding of it. Most important is deciding to do something about your drinking and implementing a plan of action.

CHAPTER 3

Self-Medication

When I tried to wash the ghosts from my head,
what I washed away was my whole life instead.
PRESTON W. LONG

In the last chapter, I reviewed the reasons why a person may develop a problem with alcohol. Some may have a genetic vulnerability to using alcohol excessively and can view themselves as having a disease. Others may view their alcohol use more as a learned behavior. No matter how you understand your problem with alcohol, you should not view yourself as a weak person, which, in my opinion, makes no sense at all.

EMOTIONS AND ALCOHOL USE

Whether you view your alcohol problem as a disease or as learned behavior, emotional or psychological concerns can be relevant to your problem as well. For example, some people may have a genetic vulnerability to developing a problem with alcohol, and they also discover that alcohol helps them relax and socialize with others. The interaction of their biological makeup and the discovery that drinking makes them feel better may help explain how the drinking problem developed. Even those without a genetic susceptibility may have learned that alcohol helps them feel less stressed, and over time they begin to rely on alcohol to relax.

The term *self-medication* is often used to explain why people drink too much. People may use alcohol to deal with stress, to decrease anxiety, and to calm down. In fact, a common belief is that individuals who use alcohol excessively must be dealing with some significant psychological issues. If they were not, then they would not be drinking so much. Those who struggle with alcohol, their loved ones, and even treatment providers often believe that people must be self-medicating some psychological pain, which then must be addressed if they are going to get better. Perhaps this reasoning resonates with your thinking: you may believe that your use of alcohol is self-medication for some type of emotional distress.

A CLOSER LOOK AT SELF-MEDICATION

I believe that the concept of self-medication is often overused and misunderstood and can, at times, interfere with the treatment of people who misuse alcohol. In this chapter, I review what self-medication is and explain why we must exercise caution when using this term to understand excessive alcohol use. Self-medicating often has nothing to do with psychological pain being the underlying cause for a drinking problem. I outline the different ways that self-medication can present, and I also explain why it is so important not to overuse this concept.

The Self-Medication Hypothesis

The term *self-medication* suggests that people use alcohol or other substances to cope with their feelings. One hypothesis has it that psychiatric illness and emotional pain are relevant to the development of an alcohol or drug use disorder. People have learned that a substance can help them feel better, such as feeling less anxious or depressed, and they are essentially playing pharmacist with themselves. They have learned that using alcohol can help them cope with some arduous life circumstance. A relapse to alcohol or other drugs may be also be triggered by painful feelings that a substance temporarily relieves.

What the Research Shows

Research has shown that there is often a relationship between psychological pain and substance use and that using substances can "help" people deal with their feelings. However, there is other research that does not support this idea or that does so only partially. In fact, I conducted some research where I asked people what factors were relevant to their relapse. While some reported that they were feeling anxious or depressed at the time of relapse, many others stated that they simply wanted to "get high."

Other research has looked at people over time to see whether having a psychiatric illness increases their chance of developing a substance use disorder. Again, although some studies have demonstrated that having a psychiatric disorder increases one's risk of developing a problem with substance use, this has not been universally demonstrated. And when a connection has been found, it is not completely clear why this occurs. It may be that other factors related to having a psychiatric disorder, such as being homeless or unemployed, lead someone to misusing alcohol as opposed to the psychiatric disorder itself. For example, homelessness can bring someone into contact with people who use drugs and alcohol and being unemployed can make someone bored, which can then lead to alcohol or drug use.

What I Have Seen

In my clinical experience, I have met many people who spoke of feeling uncomfortable in their skin and being unable to sit with their feelings, and using alcohol or another drug provided them with some short-term relief. At the same time, I have worked with others who could not come up with any reason for why they drank so much. They reported being happy with their life and having success in many areas; even so, when they started to drink, they often drank too much and didn't know why they did it.

Summary

The idea that people who drink too much are self-medicating for emotional pain is one way to understand their heavy use of alcohol and certainly may be relevant in some cases. You may even believe that this explains your use of alcohol: in some way, alcohol helps you deal with life's challenges.

IT IS ALWAYS MORE THAN JUST SELF-MEDICATION

We have learned much in recent decades about how substance use affects the brain, and an addiction to alcohol or drugs is now viewed as a brain condition. Over time, heavy use of substances makes "hardwired" changes to the brain that are responsible for the transition from recreational user to addict. These changes are also likely related to craving and relapse.

Thus, even if self-medication was, on some level, the reason why someone turned to alcohol initially and then continued to use it, other important factors are changes to the brain that resulted from the heavy use of alcohol. The person's brain gets "hijacked" by alcohol, which helps to explain that person's continued overuse. Physiological dependence on alcohol, which I review in chapter 6, may also be at work. Your body may have gotten so used to having alcohol that you now need it just to feel normal.

Painful Emotions May Not Always Be Relevant

In my career, I have had the opportunity to work on locked inpatient psychiatric units and to run therapy groups with patients who suffered from both significant psychiatric disorders and alcohol use. When I asked them what factors were relevant to their ongoing struggle with using alcohol and not achieving abstinence, they sometimes talked about dealing with challenging emotions; just as often, though, I heard stories about walking by a liquor store, seeing beer commercials on television, seeing old friends who continued to drink, or simply craving alcohol. In fact, I often heard that things were going well in their lives, yet despite that, they had relapsed. My research also supports this: when I surveyed 350 people in a substance use treatment program, one of the most common reasons they reported for relapsing was just "wanting to get high."

And Then There Are Genetics

As I explained in the last chapter, there are powerful genetic loadings that can lead someone to develop an alcohol problem. While psychological pain can be relevant, we cannot forget about underlying inherited factors. We must also remember that there are many people who suffer from serious emotional problems who do not use alcohol. They may have experimented with alcohol, but drinking never had the powerful appeal for them that it does for people who develop an alcohol use disorder. The point is that even when self-medication is germane, excessive alcohol use is more than just self-medication.

What Do You Think?

So, perhaps you believe that your use of alcohol helps you cope with some kind of stress or emotional difficulties. While that may be true, it is important for you to appreciate that using alcohol to handle your emotions is only one piece of the puzzle. In addition, an addiction to alcohol use has taken hold of your life and affected your brain, which also contributes to your drinking problem. Even if your problems went away, you would likely still be tempted to drink and might find yourself drinking too much.

IS SELF-MEDICATION STILL RELEVANT?

As I admitted above, it is possible that when some people first began to drink, they discovered that alcohol helped them cope in some way with the challenges of life. Some may have discovered that alcohol relieved their social anxiety and made them more comfortable in group situations. Others may have learned that when they drank, they were able to forget, at least temporarily, some painful memories from the past. We could say these people were self-medicating to cope with life, but we must also ask whether this reason continues to account for their ongoing drinking.

For example, Joe, a 42-year-old married man whom I saw for his ongoing struggles with alcohol (he had just been arrested for driving under the influence of alcohol), told me that he first began to use alcohol to fit in with his peer group in high school. In college, too, he struggled with some self-consciousness and social anxiety and continued to cope with these emotions by drinking. When I asked him if he still struggled with social anxiety, he said he generally felt comfortable in most social situations, although he would drink to relax. He truly did not know whether he continued to struggle with social anxiety because he always drank in those situations.

I suggested to him that I first wanted to help him stop his alcohol use, and then we could see how he felt after he'd stopped. What Joe found out was that after he stopped drinking, he was not a particularly anxious man and was able to be in social situations without difficulty. He did struggle with abstaining from alcohol, but it had nothing to do with any social anxiety he felt. The point is that while self-medication may have initiated Joe's drinking, years later he first had to stop drinking before he even realized that his old reason no longer pertained.

What Do You Think?

Maybe you can relate to Joe. When you first began to drink many years ago, it may have helped in some ways, but currently those reasons may no longer be relevant. Consider a person who began to smoke cigarettes as a teenager to feel a part of a peer group. Now, wanting to fit in has nothing to do with why the adult continues to smoke. Instead, smoking cigarettes has become an addiction, which explains why the person continues to smoke. Maybe your use of alcohol fulfilled a need when you first began to drink, but currently your original reasons for drinking may no longer exist.

BELIEVING IN SELF-MEDICATION
TO TAKE THE FOCUS OFF OF ALCOHOL

I have worked with many people struggling with their use of alcohol who report that they use alcohol to relieve their unwanted feelings. They may mention the stress of their job, their marital problems, or the challenges of dealing with their children. While these concerns are undeniably real, they want to view their excessive use of alcohol as being caused by their life's difficulties; it gives them a parsimonious explanation for why they drink so much. People want to understand why they do certain things, and it is common to attribute drinking to some pressing external factor. Furthermore, they may believe that if they could only solve those problems, their drinking problem might resolve itself. Viewing their life's difficulties as the cause of their drinking can help take the focus off their drinking and minimize the severity of their drinking problem.

An example of this is Mary, who at the age of 56 ended up in the hospital for acute pancreatitis secondary to her drinking. She told me that she had been drinking too much, which she attributed to having lost both of her parents in the past two years. While Mary's understanding of her drinking made intuitive sense and was quite compelling, a review of her past treatment records revealed that she had been admitted to the hospital about five years ago after a fall related to her drinking. Her husband also reported that she had been drinking problematically for many years. Although his wife was upset about the loss of her parents, he felt that her drinking had nothing to do with that, as it had been excessive long before they died.

In summary, there may be times when self-medication appears to explain a drinking problem for someone who reports that painful feelings are the cause for drinking. However, with further review, that person's belief in self-medication is more of a way to justify drinking. It can also be a means of minimizing the severity of the problem by offering the hope that, if the problems only went away, so too would the problem with drinking.

What Do You Think?

Have you fallen into this trap, just like Mary? Do you justify your drinking by thinking that your life stress is causing your drinking problem? While your drinking may help you manage some life stress, or at least you think it does, did your drinking problem actually precede whatever struggles you now have? Is it possible that the problems you have in your life and your drinking have become fused in your mind so that you use those problems to justify your drinking? Being honest with yourself is paramount when answering these questions.

SELF-MEDICATING THE PAINFUL EMOTIONS CAUSED BY ALCOHOL USE

There are also times when people who struggle with alcohol believe that the emotional pain they experience is what causes their drinking. They maintain that they are alleviating their pain by drinking. However, *the primary suffering they are experiencing has been caused by their drinking.* That is, their painful feelings did not cause their alcohol use in a true etiological sense. In fact, when their drinking problem had developed, they seemed to be functioning well and were generally happy. However, over time, as their alcohol problem worsened and they experienced problems secondary to their misuse of alcohol, they began to believe that these problems were the cause of their drinking.

I am reminded of Ken, a 60-year-old divorced man with two adult children. I saw Ken when he was in an inpatient detoxification program. Ken was very depressed about his life. Not only did his marriage end in divorce about three years before I met him, but during the past year, he told me that his children, too, had distanced themselves from him. He was feeling very isolated and lonely, and he stated that his use of alcohol helped him cope with his terrible life circumstances and the losses he had experienced.

As I explored with him why his marriage had ended as well as why his children had distanced themselves from him, he told me that he had lost his job about six years ago and found it difficult to find another one. This, in turn, caused much financial stress and friction in his marriage, which he noted was a big reason why his wife left him. He also reported that his children were always closer with his wife and that, after the divorce, they tended to side with her. He was feeling very depressed and drank to cope.

Although Ken's story was compelling, I later had an opportunity to meet his ex-wife and children, something that Ken agreed to, as he thought it would be a good idea. Their story was strikingly different from his: according to his ex-wife, the reason he had lost his job and could not find another one was that he drank too much. She also stated that she divorced him because of his drinking. His children told a similar story: they decided to withdraw from him as they could not tolerate his drinking, and for their own well-being, they needed to detach from him. Although these losses were painful for Ken, they were not the underlying reasons for his drinking. *Rather, his drinking caused these problems, although Ken came to believe that these problems caused his drinking.* He was self-medicating the pain that was due to his drinking.

What Do You Think?

Think about yourself and your drinking. Has your drinking caused you problems, and do you use these difficulties to explain your drinking? Is it possible that many, if not most, of the problems you experience have been caused by your drinking instead of those problems being the reason why you drink? Again, honesty with yourself is of utmost importance.

WHY IS THIS IMPORTANT FOR YOU?

What does it matter how you view the relationship between your emotional challenges and your use of alcohol? What difference does it make if you want to think that your life problems are responsible for your drinking? It is important because viewing your alcohol problem as being caused by something else can shift your focus away from your drinking problem and toward other things, which may lead you to continue to drink in unhealthy ways.

The truth is that regardless of the relationship between your drinking and your other life problems, if you are going to get better, it is critical that you focus on your drinking as a problem in and of itself. *If previous or current difficulties in life have caused and are causing you, at least in part, to self-medicate with alcohol in unhealthy ways, you need to get help for those problems, but at the same time, you must also address your drinking.*

Emotional Pain Is No Reason to Drink

You should not think that you must address your emotional concerns prior to doing something about your drinking. *Even if your drinking is due to severe problems in your life, continuing to use alcohol to cope will only make your problems worse, as your drinking will add further insult to whatever you are struggling with. You need to work simultaneously on both your problem with alcohol and your other problems.*

Both Problems Need Equal Attention

It is not as though your emotional problems are primary and your alcohol problem is secondary. *Regardless of what problem came first, now both issues are primary, and both need equal attention.* Allowing your reasons for drinking to justify continuing to drink will only keep you stuck where you are. Whatever your justifications for drinking are, you must learn to manage them in healthier ways because drinking is not a solution.

SUMMARY

Whether you view your drinking as a learned behavior, a disease, or a combination of the two, emotional problems often get tied to drinking. Self-medication could explain, at least in part, how your alcohol problem originally developed. However, there are other ways that psychological pain and alcohol get entwined that have nothing to do with emotional pain being the cause of your drinking. In fact, there are times when painful feelings do not cause the drinking but instead are caused by it.

Whatever the relationship between your emotions and drinking, you should not think that you must address your psychological problems before you address your drinking problem or that, in order to resolve your drinking, you must resolve your other problems. This is not to say that your emotional concerns are not relevant. They need to be attended to, *but you must also put a plan in place to address your drinking. Continuing to drink to cope will never work. Not only will this prevent you from learning other ways to manage your problems, but continued drinking will also cause you further problems.*

The bottom line is that there is no reason—good, bad, or otherwise—to continue to use alcohol to deal with your problems. Drinking will only make your entire situation worse.

PART II

Before You
Get Started

CHAPTER 4

Getting Ready and Staying Motivated

A person with half volition goes backwards and forwards,
but makes no progress on even the smoothest of roads.
THOMAS CARLYLE

It's not that some people have willpower and some don't.
It's that some people are ready to change and others are not.
JAMES GORDON, MD

Things do not change. We change.
HENRY DAVID THOREAU

By now you have enough information to know that you have a problem with alcohol. You have honestly evaluated your situation and
have reached the conclusion that your use of alcohol is causing you
difficulty in one or more areas of your life. You may also have given a
name to your problem with alcohol, whether you call it a disease or a
bad habit. And you have learned that you should not beat yourself up
for having an alcohol problem or blame your drinking on any psychological problems, though they may be relevant. You are no different
from the person who struggles in other ways, such as an individual
who can't always control his or her temper, stress level, or tendency
to work too much. Things are somewhat out of your control, and you
are stuck in a pattern of behavior that is causing you distress. However, that happens to most people in some way during the course of
their life.

As I stated in the first chapter, while it is difficult to look at your drinking and arrive at the realization that your use of alcohol is a problem, it is often even more difficult to make the decision to change your pattern of alcohol use and put a plan into action. You enjoy many things about drinking despite the fact that drinking also hurts you. You may enjoy how drinking makes you feel, the social aspects of drinking, the way it relaxes you, the taste, or the fun it provides you. At the same time, you may occasionally not like how you act when you drink too much or how drinking negatively affects your relationship with your wife, husband, girlfriend, or boyfriend; how it hurts you financially; or how drinking too much makes you feel bad the next day. However, not wanting to give up the positive aspects of drinking can make it hard to take action, can make you question your decision to change, and can play a role in leading you back to your old behaviors.

AMBIVALENCE

Ambivalence is having simultaneous and contradictory feelings or attitudes toward something, whether this is a person, object, or action. And this can lead to uncertainty about what course of action to take. As a result, movement doesn't occur, and you stay the present course. Ambivalence can keep a person stuck.

You should know that ambivalence is different from not acknowledging that you have a problem. You may fully realize that drinking is a problem for you, yet you may not have made the decision to take action and change your relationship to alcohol. I have worked with many people who knew that their use of alcohol was a problem but were not ready to do the work to change their behavior. I have often heard things like this:

- "I am drinking too much, but I am not sure if I am ready to stop."

- "I don't know what to do. I know my drinking is hurting me, but I like it, too."

- "Boy, I know my drinking is damaging my relationship with my wife, but I enjoy drinking with my friends and don't know what I would do if I couldn't party with them."

- "Drinking is my downfall, but it is also my best friend."

- "I wish I would want to change. I know drinking is bad for me, but I just can't get up the desire to do something different and really change. I wish there was some kind of magic pill that I could take!"

Ambivalence can also lead you to slip back into your old ways. Mixed feelings can make you question yourself: "Why am I doing this?" "Do I really want to be doing this?" "Do I really want to change?" I have certainly seen people who have made the decision to address their drinking problem but for whom, at some point, something changes. Their commitment begins to waver, and they start to question themselves and their decision. For example, after deciding to quit drinking and successfully not drinking for several weeks, they may lose their commitment and start up again.

Ambivalence Is Universal

It is common for people to know that they have a problem but not be ready to change, or after having made a decision to change, they lose their commitment and resume their old behaviors. For example, many people are overweight and realize that they need to lose weight but aren't ready to take the steps to begin a diet. They may not like the way they feel, their doctors may have recommended that they lose weight, and they may not like the way they look. However, they love to eat and obtain many positive benefits from eating. They don't want to give up their favorite foods, eat less, or lose the social aspects of eating. Despite the negative consequences of eating too much and being overweight, they fail to commit to action and change their eating habits. Or they begin a diet that starts well, but at some point they go off it and resume their out-of-control eating.

And what about cigarette smokers who know well the dangers of smoking, can list many reasons for wanting to quit, and yet don't commit to stop smoking? Why don't they just stop? Apart from the physical withdrawal that can occur when someone stops smoking, there may be many other reasons for continuing to smoke, whether it is the relaxation that smoking provides, the enjoyment of smoking, or even the fear of withdrawal, to name just a few factors that can prevent someone from taking action. There are also smokers who joke, "It is easy to quit smoking. I have done it a dozen times!" These people made the decision to stop smoking, but at some point their motivation faded away and they returned to smoking.

There are also people who are in a difficult relationship and just can't decide whether they should leave their partner. While they may be very unhappy and can list numerous things they don't like about the person they're with, they also see positive aspects of staying the present course. They may like some things about their partner, or perhaps there are financial reasons for staying together. Their ambivalent feelings prevent them from taking action and keep them stuck. Some end up in a "ping-pong" type of relationship, breaking up and getting back together every few months on account of their mixed feelings.

For some people, ambivalence results from a fear of changing and doing something different. While a part of them wants to change, and they can see benefits to changing, another part of them is too scared to take an unfamiliar path—such as living life without alcohol. So they remain the same and never quite get around to putting a plan of action into place.

Coming to Terms with Ambivalence

To develop and sustain a plan of action to change your behavior, you must do several things:

- You must overcome ambivalence.

- You must put an action plan into place.

- You must stay on course.

Resolving ambivalence is absolutely essential if you are going to change your pattern of drinking. And the first step is to *become certain and remain certain* that the bad consequences of your drinking outweigh the advantages, or that the benefits of changing appeal to you more than the drawbacks of changing. Whatever thrusts you into and keeps you on a course of action, the need to change must become and remain more important than staying the same.

WHAT ARE YOUR "BECAUSES"?

I often tell my patients that they must become crystal clear about their "becauses," and you need to be clear about them as well. What I mean is that you are thinking about changing your relationship to alcohol *because* your use of alcohol is either hurting you a lot or preventing you from getting what you want out of life. Your decision to change your use of alcohol may have nothing to do with your no longer wanting to drink. You like to drink! In the best of all worlds, you would continue to drink and not even think about drinking differently. There must be powerful reasons you must remember that are driving you to change your pattern of drinking, and you must always remain mindful of them. This will help you to stay the course and resolve any ambivalence you have about changing.

Although Consequences Are Important, You Need a Vision

I have worked with many people who have experienced significant negative consequences from drinking, yet they have continued to drink and have continued to experience severe repercussions. They have not completely come to terms with their ambivalence about changing their use of alcohol.

What I have discovered is that, often, they are fully aware of the consequences of their drinking, but they do not have a vision for themselves of how their life could change in a positive way if they addressed their drinking. Consequences are simply not that important when you lack a vision of what your life could be like or how better life could be without drinking. I strongly encourage you to think not only about how your drinking has hurt you but also about what positive things can occur if you resolve your drinking problem. Remaining mindful of the benefits that can come from resolving your problem with alcohol will help you overcome any ambivalence you may have.

Complete the Exercises

The exercise I call "Pros and Cons of My Drinking" on page 77 can help you come to terms with your ambivalence. Think carefully about what you like and don't like about your drinking. How does drinking help you, and how does drinking hurt you? Focus on your social life, your health, your financial situation, your work, your important relationships, any legal problems drinking may have caused you, and your self-esteem and emotional well-being. How does drinking impact any of these things, both in positive and negative ways?

Next, complete the "Pros and Cons of My Changing" exercise on page 77. Think about the advantages that changing your relationship to alcohol will offer, and also think about the disadvantages of changing your drinking pattern. While there may be some overlap with the previous exercise, there can be some important differences, as the case of Mike shows.

Mike's drinking had for years had a negative impact on his relationship with Nancy, his wife. Over the years, Mike and Nancy had had numerous arguments about his drinking, but no screaming or pleading by Nancy about Mike's drinking ever made a difference. Mike primarily came to see me to placate Nancy. He knew his drinking was problematic, but he wasn't sure whether he was truly ready to change it. He knew his drinking was destroying his marriage but seemed to accept this and couldn't come up with any other harm that resulted from his drinking.

I asked Mike to complete the Pros and Cons of My Drinking exercise. He wrote down a number of pros, including

- "socializing with my friends"
- "relaxing"
- "love partying"

For cons, the only thing he could come up with was

- "hurts my marriage"

Mike next completed the Pros and Cons of My Changing exercise, and the first thing he wrote under pros was

- "could get along with my wife and have fun again"

At that moment, I noticed a change in his demeanor and attitude, and I asked him about it. Mike said that, while he had always known that his drinking caused arguments between him and Nancy, he hadn't ever thought much about how he could have a loving relationship with Nancy if he stopped drinking. That point, which should have been self-evident, somehow got lost in all of their arguing. Mike was flabbergasted by this realization, and it was the deciding factor that motivated him to change his pattern of drinking. For Mike, a perceived benefit of changing was a greater motivator than was a negative consequence of his drinking.

After completing these exercises, read each item you wrote, and think about how important the particular drawbacks and benefits are for you. Focus on each reason until you have a clear sense of how important it is. On a scale of 1 to 10, with 1 being very unimportant and 10 being very important, rank each item to see what reasons are most important to you. Often it is not the total number of reasons in a particular category that can help you determine whether you are ready to change, but rather one or more reasons will really stick out to you as essential. Mike didn't even need to rank each of his reasons—he came to see what was most important to him spontaneously. This was not true for John.

John was a 38-year-old married man, the father of 7- and 10-year-old boys. In retrospect, he had had a drinking problem since his early twenties. He drank on most days, which caused daily arguments with his wife. He reported that this was affecting their relationship, and their yelling matches caused a lot of tension in the home. On the weekends, John drank more heavily, so much so that often an entire Sunday was blown as he slept off his hangover. John came to see me after he was arrested for drunk driving.

John admitted that he drank a fair amount and that drinking might be a problem for him, but he generally minimized the degree to which it caused him problems and affected his family. He understood his recent arrest as a case of being in the wrong place at the wrong time, but he also acknowledged that he often drove drunk and that this wasn't the best idea. He wasn't sure whether he was ready to change his relationship with alcohol.

I observed that John seemed to have some mixed feelings, and I asked him if he would complete the Pros and Cons of My Drinking and Pros and Cons of My Changing exercises. On the first exercise, he wrote down many pros, including

- "seeing my friends"
- "It's fun."
- "I like the feeling."
- "I like the taste of beer."
- "It helps me unwind."
- "I like the social scene."

The only cons he could come up with were

- "getting arrested"
- "wife problems"

On the Pros and Cons of My Changing exercise, the only pros John wrote were

- "won't ever get arrested again"
- "My wife would give me less grief."

He came up with many cons of changing, including

- "boredom"
- "not being able to see my friends"
- "missing the bar scene"
- "wouldn't be able to have fun"
- "couldn't unwind"

Before going through his list to see what was most important to him, I wanted John to be sure to cover all of the possible pros and cons. It seemed to me that some important things might be missing from his list—for example, there was nothing about his health or his children. I asked him about this, and with some exploration, he was able to acknowledge that his drinking was affecting his relationship with his children. He then wrote down under the cons of his drinking

- "kids being afraid of me when I fight with my wife"
- "missing their hockey games on Sundays"

When I asked him if there would be any benefits to changing, he wrote

- "could have fun with my boys and see their hockey games"
- "kids wouldn't be afraid of me"

I then had John rank each item on his lists by order of importance. What he found was that all of the reasons that concerned his children were most important to him. While there were more reasons listed under the pros of drinking and the cons of changing, how his drinking hurt his relationship with his sons and how changing could improve their relationship led John to decide to change his pattern of drinking.

After you complete the exercise, review it *daily*. This will help you stay focused on the problems your drinking has caused you and the positive things you will gain by changing your relationship to alcohol. It will reinforce your initial commitment to change and keep your motivation going.

Mixed Feelings Don't Just Evaporate

Most decisions we make in life aren't black or white. Even when we make a decision, some lingering mixed feelings are to be expected. For example, think about when you have ended a relationship or changed your job. While there are times when this decision is easy and clear, there are other times when you need to weigh the advantages and disadvantages of making a switch, and the decision is harder to make. However, at some point, the scales tip, and although you may still have some mixed feelings, you are able to make a decision.

The reasons and feelings that could keep you from putting an action plan into place or that could creep back into your mind and make you doubt your decision—the pros of drinking and the cons of changing—don't simply go away. *They can persist, but despite this, you can move forward anyway.*

Focus on the negative aspects of your drinking and the positive things you can get by changing, as opposed to the benefits of your drinking or the negative things about changing. The goal is for you to realize that the reasons for changing outweigh and are more important to you than continuing to drink the way you have been.

Are You Still Not Sure?

After completing the two exercises, you may find that the advantages of changing and the harmful consequences of your drinking don't outweigh the advantages of drinking and the disadvantages of changing. Or you may see the need for change but may be scared to address your drinking, so much so that your fear prevents you from taking action. While you know that drinking is hurting you, there are things about drinking that you can't imagine not having, and these stop you from taking action. Maybe your ambivalence hasn't yet been resolved. You may still be thinking about changing and aren't yet ready to take control of your life and your drinking problem.

If you aren't sure whether the cons of drinking and the pros of changing outweigh the pros of drinking and the cons of changing . . .

- Make the commitment to change for a limited period of time to see what it is like. If you don't like it, you can always go back to the way you were. Thus, you have little to lose but much potentially to gain. You owe it to yourself to at least experience something different, which may help you make a longer-term decision. I am sure that you will find your life gets better once your drinking problem has been resolved.

If you are afraid to change your pattern of drinking . . .

- Remember that thinking about changing is scarier than actually doing it. In fact, this book will help you manage any fear you have, if that is a stumbling block. Don't let fear stand in your way. You will find that, when the time comes, you will be able to manage the things that once concerned you the most.

If you are thinking about forever, don't. Think only about now!

- Don't think that you can never again drink the way you were drinking and how your life will be affected by that. Think only about today, stay in the present, and do not allow yourself to get overwhelmed about the future. Remember that weeks and months from now, you will think differently about your drinking than you do today. Just focus on the present and how you wish to change your pattern of drinking right now and for the present day only. Worry about tomorrow when tomorrow comes.

TWO OTHER MOTIVATION KILLERS

A Lack of Confidence and Learned Helplessness

It may be that you haven't begun the process of changing and taking action because you don't have the confidence in yourself to change. As much as you want to be different, you don't believe in yourself and your ability to make a change, so you simply don't try. You have gotten the idea that you can't change because you previously tried to change and failed. As a result, you have resigned yourself to the fact that change is not possible. Believing, without proof and evidence, that you can't succeed has been called *learned helplessness.*

Learned helplessness has been documented in research using animals. In the original experiment, dogs were placed in a box and shocked, and the only way they could escape the shock was to jump over a barrier. After repeated shocks, the dogs learned to jump over the barrier. However, dogs placed in a box that couldn't escape getting shocked couldn't even be trained to avoid shock when escape was later made possible. Instead, they gave up and accepted the shock because they had previously learned there was nothing they could do to avoid it. They had *learned* that they were helpless.

This often happens with people who struggle with alcohol consumption. After many unsuccessful attempts to quit drinking, they eventually give up, accept failure, and stop trying. They, too, have learned to be helpless.

Fortunately, the story of the helpless dogs doesn't end here. In another experiment, dogs that had accepted their fate and wouldn't escape the shock were finally trained to avoid it by being coaxed and forced by the researchers. After they were repeatedly pulled with a leash over the barrier while being shocked, the dogs eventually learned on their own to avoid the shock. With some outside prodding, they understood that they had control over their situation and were no longer helpless.

If a lack of confidence is stopping you . . .

- If you no longer believe that you can succeed, and learned helplessness plays a role in your inability to stop drinking, remember that past failure doesn't mean future failure. Don't allow the belief that you can't achieve success to become a self-fulfilling prophecy. Maybe you didn't go about it in the right way last time; learn from this rather than seeing yourself as someone who cannot change. Rarely has a person been completely successful in their first attempt to change, and this is particularly true for people who are trying to change their pattern of drinking. The dogs in the experiment learned that they could change, and you, too, need to remember that change is always possible. The key is never to give up.

A Fear of Failing

Perhaps you do not want to risk failing, so you never put an action plan into place. Or if you've failed in the past, you are all too familiar with the disappointment of not succeeding and don't want to experience that again. So instead of trying and possibly having to face failure, you stay the present course.

If a fear of failing is stopping you . . .

- Stop viewing your past attempts to get a handle on your drinking as failures. Instead, see them as unsuccessful attempts and recognize that you simply haven't succeeded yet. Failure is an end point and only happens when you stop trying. So, if you continue to try, it can never be said that you failed. You just haven't succeeded . . . *yet*.

Moving Forward

I hope, though, that you are not in any of these positions. You are reading this book, which means that you are concerned about your drinking and are seriously thinking of doing something about it. Try to keep your mind focused on the consequences of your drinking and the benefits of changing, which will help you to stay on track.

SUMMARY

Getting ready to address your drinking and staying motivated are key to your success. However, having some mixed feelings can interfere with your commitment to change. To carry through with your plan, remember to stay focused on the negative effects of your drinking and the positive things that will happen by changing your relationship to alcohol. Despite having ambivalence, you can still go forward when you keep these thoughts in mind.

If you are still feeling stuck and not committed to changing, try to accept that and commit to changing for a brief period of time to see what it is like. You can always go back to what you were doing if things do not get better for you. And if the fear of changing is stopping you, remember that the fear of doing something is always scarier than actually doing it. You will likely find that changing is not as fearful as you imagined, and within a short time, you will feel much different. And don't think about forever, which is overwhelming. Just focus on changing for the day you are living now.

Finally, try not to let a lack of confidence or a fear of failing stop you. Because you have not succeeded in the past has nothing to do with your present effort. When doing something difficult, people rarely succeed on their first try. You need to learn from past attempts, incorporate that knowledge going forward, and believe in yourself.

There are risks and costs to a program of action,
but they are far less than the long-range risks
and costs of comfortable inaction.
JOHN F. KENNEDY

Do the thing you fear to do and keep on doing it . . .
that is the quickest and surest way ever yet
discovered to conquer fear.
DALE CARNEGIE

*If you have no confidence in self, you are twice defeated
in the race of life. With confidence, you have won
even before you have started.*

MARCUS GARVEY

*I am not judged by the number of times I fail, but by the
number of times I succeed; and the number of times
I succeed is in direct proportion to the number of times
I can fail and keep on trying.*

TOM HOPKINS

Pros and Cons of My Drinking

PROS OF MY DRINKING

Write down all of the things you like about drinking—think of your relationships, your emotional state, your social life, or anything else you like about drinking. When done, rank each item 1–10, **with 1 being the least important and 10 being the most important.**

CONS OF MY DRINKING

Write down all of the ways your drinking hurts you—think of your relationships, your health, your emotional state, your job or school, your finances, or any legal troubles. When done, rank each item 1–10, **with 1 being the least important and 10 being the most important.**

Pros and Cons of My Changing

PROS OF MY CHANGING

Write down all of the ways that changing your drinking pattern may help you—think of your relationships, your health, your emotional state, your job or school, your finances, or any legal troubles. When done, rank each item 1–10, **with 1 being the least important and 10 being the most important.**

CONS OF MY CHANGING

Write down all of the ways that changing your drinking pattern may hurt you—think of your relationships, your emotional state, your social life, or any other thing that concerns you about changing your pattern of drinking. When done, rank each item 1–10, **with 1 being the least important and 10 being the most important.**

CHAPTER 5

Can You Really Help Yourself?

Only I can change my life. No one can do it for me.
CAROL BURNETT

It is the truth we ourselves speak rather than
the treatment we receive that heals us.
HOBART MOWRER

By now, you have honestly evaluated your situation and have decided that you must change your relationship to alcohol in order to lead a more fulfilling life, one free from alcohol-related problems. You have a vision for yourself, and if you continue to allow alcohol to harm your life, you will not reach your dreams. The scales have tipped in favor of changing, and you are ready to develop a plan of action.

Yet quitting or cutting down is often difficult. Perhaps you have tried before—perhaps many times, or with treatment—only to return to your old ways. Having been unable to succeed, you may feel hopeless, dejected, frustrated, and angry.

On the other hand, perhaps this is the first time that you have been serious about doing something about your drinking. Regardless of your particular situation, you may be wondering what you can do to help yourself and whether you need to seek help such as AA meetings or substance use counseling.

SOME PEOPLE THINK THAT
TREATMENT IS ESSENTIAL

Our society perpetuates the idea that no one's alcohol problem will go away without the support of a counselor, a treatment program, or a support group like AA. Advertisements for addiction treatment programs often assert that professional help is required. Statements such as "alcoholism is a treatable illness" or "alcohol problems do not go away if left untreated" dominate the social scene. In 1993, the former director of the National Institute on Drug Abuse, Robert Dupont, wrote, "Addiction is not self-curing. Left alone addiction only gets worse, leading to total degradation, to prison, and ultimately to death." Also, as I discussed in chapter 2, the idea that a drinking problem is a disease is embraced by many people. If this is true, it follows that this disease requires treatment like other diseases.

These advertisements or the idea that a drinking problem is a disease may have caused you to think that no one with a drinking problem can possibly change his or her life without receiving treatment. We all know people—family, friends, and neighbors—who have tried unsuccessfully to stop drinking on their own, which could discourage you. Or you may believe or hear from others that unless people get involved in treatment, they are not really serious about helping themselves. You may also know people who have gone to treatment and who have relapsed, which can make you think that an alcohol problem is so challenging that even with treatment, success is hard to achieve. How could people possibly do it on their own?

THE TRUTH ABOUT TREATMENT

Many, many individuals with a long history of alcohol misuse have resolved their drinking problem without attending AA or any other type of self-help meetings or without ever receiving treatment from a therapist, counselor, or treatment program of any kind. Despite a societal belief that people with an alcohol problem must obtain treatment, it is clear that even individuals who struggle with a severe alcohol problem can achieve recovery without treatment. The respected American Psychiatric Association and the Institute of Medicine state this as well.

WHAT RESEARCH SHOWS

During the past 50 years, there have been many reports of people who helped themselves with their drinking problem without treatment, either by abstaining from alcohol or by moderating their drinking. The first reports were generally cases of individuals who were able to do so. However, as research in this area has grown, studies have looked at larger populations of people. Some researchers studied people over time to see how alcohol problems progress with and without treatment; other researchers surveyed people to discover if they had a drinking problem, if they had resolved it, and if so, how.

Observing People over Time

Did people who received treatment for their drinking problem fare better over time than people who did not? Interestingly one study found that there was essentially no difference in outcomes between the groups. Regardless of whether people received treatment, the same percentage got better each year. People seemed to heal themselves, as opposed to treatment being the deciding factor.

Surveys

Surveys that ask people whether they have ever suffered from an alcohol problem and how they resolved it have also found that many people with an alcohol problem are able to help themselves. One study asked more than 11,000 people about their drinking to determine their past and present use of alcohol. Of those who said they had resolved their problem for at least one year, 75 percent reported doing it without any kind of outside help or treatment.

Another study, sponsored by the National Institute on Alcohol Abuse and Alcoholism and called the National Longitudinal Alcohol Epidemiologic Study, reported the results of interviews conducted with almost 43,000 adults over age 18 who lived throughout the United States. A lot of information was obtained, including about their alcohol use and related problems and any treatment they had received. Of the people interviewed, about 4,600 people had experienced a serious alcohol problem anywhere from 1 to 20 years before the interview.

Of those 4,600 people, about 25 percent had received treatment, and about 75 percent never received any type of treatment. Of the people who never received treatment of any kind, 74 percent were able to recover from their drinking problem.

DON'T SOME PEOPLE NEED TREATMENT?

Yes—there are two situations in which treatment is essential. Some people must be medically detoxified from their use of alcohol. As you will read in the next chapter, it can be extremely dangerous for someone who is physiologically dependent on alcohol to stop drinking suddenly without professional assistance. Other people who have a drinking problem have additional serious difficulties in their lives, which can interfere with their ability to go it alone. These problems may include depression, unemployment and related stress, domestic violence, marital breakup, legal challenges, and others. People who drink alcohol excessively with serious social or emotional difficulties will have more trouble getting a handle on their alcohol use without treatment and some kind of outside support. Such individuals should seek the help and guidance of trained substance use disorder professionals.

However, even for people who need or want treatment, what they bring to it and their internal motivation and desire to change are critical for their success. Without commitment and hard work, treatment won't do much.

YOU CAN AND MUST HELP YOURSELF

The idea that the majority of people who struggle with alcohol consumption are able to help themselves without treatment fits with my experience. I have found that treatment is often the least important factor when a person resolves a drinking problem.

Over the years, I have spoken with numerous individuals with a serious alcohol problem who had been admitted many times for detoxification to inpatient alcoholism treatment programs. Typically, shortly after being discharged, they began to drink again, and within a fairly short period of time, they needed to be admitted once again. However, after being discharged one particular time, they remained abstinent. They were not sure what was different, but something had "clicked." They finally were ready to get serious about ending their problem with alcohol. Whatever triggered the change, they had had enough.

As we talked, I was struck with how, at that moment of their decision, their mental state, not the treatment, had been the most important factor. It is even possible that, at that time, they would have achieved success without treatment simply because they were ready to change their life.

Suzie was a 59-year-old woman who had been abstinent from alcohol for the past 13 years. Suzie began drinking in her teenage years, and rather quickly, alcohol took over her life. In fact, by her report, drinking was her life. From her late twenties until she stopped drinking, she spent as much time in various treatment programs as out of them. She couldn't remember how many times she had been in the hospital for detoxification but guessed it must be at least 50. When

Suzie drank, she would often become suicidal, and on numerous occasions, she was admitted to a psychiatric hospital to keep her safe. Suzie became known as a "frequent flyer" because of the number of times she was admitted to the hospital. Both Suzie and the staff came to believe that she probably would never stop drinking.

But Suzie did finally stop drinking. During one admission (her last), she made the decision that she had to change her life. After her detoxification, she went into a longer-term residential program, graduated from it, and never returned to drinking. In fact, Suzie started working at a residential treatment program for people who struggle with substance abuse.

Through my work, I met Suzie and learned of her history of alcohol problems. I was very interested in how she had been able to stop drinking after years of being unable to. What finally did it for her? Was it a counselor she saw or the residential treatment program she got involved in? Maybe it was AA? Did something happen in that last admission that seemed to turn her around? I asked her this, and after thinking a long time, all she could say was "I guess I was finally ready."

THERE ARE NO MAGIC BULLETS

A treatment program will not end your problem with alcohol consumption. It is you who must make the decision and make the change. While treatment is often critical for those who need additional help and support, for many people treatment is almost the least important variable. As the saying goes, "you can lead a horse to water, but you can't make it drink." Well, you can force a person into treatment, but unless the person is ready to do something about the problem, treatment will generally not be successful. And this is not a put-down for treatment. While treatment can sometimes help increase a person's motivation to change, be a catalyst for a person to begin a change effort, and provide a chance for an individual to see what life is like without being under the influence of alcohol, it can only do so much. The point is that treatment is no magic bullet. *You are the key and most important ingredient!*

A lot of research has tried to understand what is responsible for successful behavioral change when a person sees a therapist, regardless of the type of problem the person is struggling with. What makes treatment work, and what is responsible for treatment going well? It should be no surprise to you that, regardless of the specific problem, the most important factor when a person tries to change is the person him- or herself. While having a good social support network is important, your readiness, motivation, and acceptance of personal responsibility to change are essential.

THE RIGHT ATTITUDE

Again, if you do not have serious psychiatric or other problems, you may be able to help yourself without professional help or attendance at group support meetings. What will help? Some former problem drinkers who resolved their problem report that they had "the right attitude" or that they were ready. However, to say that all it takes is the right attitude and a readiness to change isn't particularly helpful. Many problem drinkers truly want to quit, but for one reason or another, they have failed over and over again. So what makes it work when it works?

There is one thing we know. You can definitely succeed at resolving your drinking habit even if you have failed before.

Maintaining the Right Attitude

To achieve success, you need to maintain a good attitude. Otherwise there is no way you will be able to cope with the ups and downs you experience as you try to limit alcohol in your life. The right attitude consists of

- *making an intense commitment to change your life.* You need to realize that gaining control over your alcohol consumption is something that you have to do. Changing your relationship to alcohol must become a major life priority and must at least for some time be on the front burner. Take responsibility for your drinking and remain committed to changing your use of alcohol.

- *remembering the problems that drinking has caused you (and will cause you) and no longer wanting to deal with those problems.* Without wallowing in the pain related to your past drinking, maintain a clear understanding of the harm you will again experience if you lapse into your old ways. Make the decision to change your pattern of drinking so that you will never experience this pain again.

- *keeping in mind how you want your life to be and remembering that unless you get control of your drinking, you will never achieve that.* Remember what you want your life to look like and that you must change your pattern of drinking if you are going to realize your dreams and get what you want out of life. Never forget that your old pattern of drinking will prevent you from attaining your goals.

- *finding joy in your life without excessive drinking and never wanting to lose that happiness.* You must work hard to enjoy your life without alcohol. Learn to enjoy life every bit as much, if not more, despite drinking less or not at all. And remember that if you return to uncontrolled drinking, you will lose that happiness and your life will be worse.

- *learning to cope with problems without using alcohol.* Even though you may often feel like drinking, you must deal with your problems without drinking or without drinking excessively. No matter what, drinking to cope can't be an option.

In other words, while you may need to develop new skills and habits, your attitude is more crucial than a treatment program. When you have these five components of the right attitude, along with the development of certain skills, you will be able to achieve success.

IF PEOPLE CAN HELP THEMSELVES,
WHY IS THERE OUTSIDE HELP?

If people can help themselves with their drinking problem, why are professional treatment and self-help groups available? Treatment programs exist because some people find that despite their best efforts, long-term success does not happen without outside help. Some people require objective, professional input. As was previously mentioned, this is particularly true for people who experience other serious difficulties in addition to their drinking problem. Such people may require intensive structure, safe housing, and significant support to be successful. Others may not have a social support system to help them with their drinking problem. They may have experienced a number of losses in their life because of their drinking, so the opportunity to obtain external support is essential for them to achieve success. Without treatment, some people would not succeed and would suffer severe consequences as a result of their drinking, including death.

What is more, some people find it helpful to talk things over with someone who will keep their confidence, who is nonjudgmental, who has their best interests at heart, and who can help them sort through choices and unseen obstacles. Many people find invaluable support by attending AA, other group meetings, or speaking with a professional therapist.

When you think about it, this same principle operates in other areas. To lose weight, some people want or need to involve themselves in a group program, with weekly meetings and lots of structure. Others may require only a specified diet, which they hold to faithfully. Still others go it alone by watching what they eat and changing their eating habits. As another example, let's take exercise. Some need to join a health club to institute their exercise program. There, they do group aerobics or take up swimming. Others may be able to structure their exercise regimen with exercise equipment in their home or by jogging in a park. Very simply, different people need, want, and require different input to change their life. There is no right or wrong road to success, just different routes.

Whatever route a person takes, the most important element is the person's commitment and willingness to change.

If you are going to change your relationship to alcohol, it is mostly up to you. You need to make the decision to change your life and stay focused on your goal of getting a handle on your drinking so that you and your loved ones no longer need to suffer from the harm of your drinking. No treatment program can give you that, and it is the most important ingredient for your success. And I believe this is great news because it means that you have the power and ability to change your use of alcohol.

Along with this determination, you need to work hard to enjoy your life, keep your vision of how you want your life to be in the forefront of your mind, and learn to cope with stresses, demands, and pressures without drinking. If you have or can develop these necessary beliefs and skills, you will be able to help yourself with your drinking problem. This book is designed to help you develop these skills.

On the other hand, if you experience uncontrollable emotional stress or severe depression, or you want the support of a therapist or support group, you will do better to seek some additional help at the outset. A major point to remember, though, is that whether you seek outside help or decide to tackle your drinking problem on your own, your success will be largely up to you. Your attitude, commitment, and hard work are essential.

SUMMARY

The idea that anyone who has an alcohol problem must enter a treatment program to get better permeates society. While treatment can be helpful, and for some is essential, the truth of the matter is that many people who have struggled with alcohol have resolved their problem without ever obtaining formal treatment. I believe that a person's readiness and willingness to change his or her life and relationship with alcohol is the most important variable. In fact, even among people who require treatment, their commitment to change is more important than the treatment program.

To achieve success, you must maintain the right attitude, which consists of

- making an intense commitment to change your life;

- remembering the problems that drinking has caused you (and will cause you) and no longer wanting to deal with those problems;

- keeping in mind how you want your life to be and remembering that unless you get control of your drinking, you will never achieve that;

- finding joy in your life without excessive drinking and never wanting to lose that happiness; and

- learning to cope with problems without using alcohol.

Not only can you help yourself, but you must help yourself! You are the most important factor to your success.

CHAPTER 6

You May Need Medical Help

Intelligence is knowing when you need to ask for help.
ANONYMOUS

Even people with a severe alcohol problem do not always drink every day. As a result, they may not notice any withdrawal symptoms (described below) even though their bodies may experience some toxicity as a result of their drinking. Usually, such individuals can safely stop drinking without the need for outside medical assistance. For daily drinkers who consume large quantities of alcohol, however, medically assisted detoxification is probably a necessity, although I have worked with many individuals who, despite daily and heavy drinking, did not experience a significant withdrawal syndrome when they stopped drinking. While there are exceptions, if you are a daily and heavy drinker and your body has become used to alcohol, it can be extremely dangerous for you to stop drinking suddenly without medical assistance.

ARE YOU PHYSIOLOGICALLY DEPENDENT ON ALCOHOL?

The big questions are these: How much does your body need alcohol? Without alcohol, do you experience serious bodily stress? If your system has become accustomed to alcohol, your stopping suddenly may cause serious and dangerous withdrawal symptoms:

- high blood pressure
- anxiety and tremors

- seizures

- rapid heartbeat

- increased sweating

- auditory, visual, and tactile hallucinations

- delirium

- mental confusion and agitation

- nausea and vomiting

- headache

- inability to sleep

In many cases these symptoms are few and relatively mild. In other cases they can be so severe as to cause further damage to your system. If you suffer any of these symptoms—even slightly—when you stop consuming alcohol, you need to consult a medical professional. If you need some alcohol in the morning to "stop the shakes," you require detoxification.

A severe alcohol problem needs medically supervised detoxification. If you are subject to withdrawal symptoms, medical detoxification involves replacing the alcohol in your system with another drug. This will allow you to withdraw from alcohol gradually and safely—usually over a four- or five-day period. Who will experience alcohol withdrawal symptoms? Generally, the risk of withdrawal is greater

—the more people drink, especially if they drink heavily daily;

—the more years a person has been drinking;

—for older drinkers; and

—for people who have experienced withdrawal problems in the past, even if long ago.

DRINKING CAN CAUSE OTHER MEDICAL PROBLEMS

In addition to alcohol withdrawal problems, the heavy regular use of alcohol can cause other damage for which you may need to see your doctor:

- anemia

- gastrointestinal bleeding

- liver disease

- pancreatitis

- alcoholic myopathy

- congestive heart failure

- dehydration

- cognitive and memory impairment

Any of these medical conditions may abate with abstinence, but they also can become permanent. Consequently, if you have been drinking a lot, it would be a good idea to have your doctor examine you to ensure that your medical condition is stable and that you do not have any serious health problem that requires treatment.

The safest and best action to take in preparing to quit is to see a medical doctor. It can't hurt, and you can rule out any medical problems. You will then be doing what is best for your health.

MEDICAL DETOXIFICATION: WHAT HAPPENS

The most common setting for medical detoxification is a substance use disorder treatment program with an inpatient medical detoxification service. There are also inpatient hospital programs that offer medical detoxification. These are typically geared to people who require medical intervention for serious medical concerns in addition to needing detoxification from alcohol. In these programs, you will be given medication to prevent a sudden, acute, and potentially dangerous withdrawal syndrome. Large amounts of this medication will be given to you to start with and then tapered off over the course of four or five days. This will allow your body to get used to not having alcohol in your system without placing undue stress on your physical or emotional health. During your inpatient stay, you will also receive individual and group counseling to help you remain alcohol free. Family members may also be asked to participate in your treatment.

THE TIMES ARE ALWAYS CHANGING

Significant changes have occurred and continue to occur in the treatment of alcohol problems over the past 20–30 years. In fact, our entire health care system, including the treatment of medical and mental illnesses, has changed during this time. The primary reason for this shift is the high financial cost of health care and the need to reduce it.

Inpatient hospital care is very expensive, with a one-day charge ranging from several hundred dollars to more than a thousand dollars, depending on the type of care required. As a result, many researchers have examined whether people need to be in a hospital to receive the care they need. The length of time that people need to be in the hospital has also been reevaluated.

Twenty or more years ago it was common for a person to be admitted to a hospital for detoxification and then remain in the hospital for an additional three or more weeks for extended rehabilitation, which was all covered by health insurance. The 28-day program was the standard treatment for an alcohol problem. Because of the enormous cost of a hospital stay of this length, however, insurance companies and researchers began to study whether this was necessary.

Essentially, they found that people who stayed in the hospital for 28 days did no better than those who spent a much shorter time in the hospital and then participated in structured outpatient treatment. As a result, if a person needed to go into a hospital for detoxification, insurance most likely would pay only for several days there, just long enough for medical detoxification. The person would then be discharged and referred to outpatient and community support.

However, there has been a shift once again to allowing more extended inpatient treatment for alcohol problems. This owes to parity laws for mental health and addiction, which generally prevent group health plans and health insurance issuers that cover mental health or substance use disorder treatment from offering inferior benefits for those conditions than the benefits extended to medical and surgical services. In addition, I believe the understanding that a substance use disorder is not the person's fault, but rather is similar to other chronic illnesses, has fostered a more compassionate view of people who struggle with addiction, which then led to lifting restrictions on the treatment of substance use disorders. The opioid epidemic has also precipitated more generous insurance benefits for people who are afflicted with a substance use problem.

Many of these extended inpatient treatment programs are state-supported public programs that may be free, whereas others are private programs that may be paid for by your health insurance company. You can contact your insurance company to find out your specific benefits and what programs they have contracts with, which will determine where you can go. You can also find out what, if any, deductible or copay is required of you. These types of programs are discussed in chapter 17.

DETOXIFYING WHILE LIVING AT HOME

Some people today go through medical detoxification on an outpatient basis without ever being in the hospital. Again, as a way to save money, it was reasoned that people could be safely detoxified at home and receive as an outpatient the same or similar individual and group counseling as provided in a hospital. Outpatient detoxification makes sense for those who are mostly physically and emotionally healthy, who have never had and are not in danger of having a severe alcohol withdrawal syndrome, and who have adequate social support at home. A doctor can determine whether this option is safe for you. While you are being detoxified and receiving tapering doses of medication, you will also receive counseling to help you decide on any aftercare treatment that you may need. This is likely to involve an outpatient substance use disorder treatment program.

SUMMARY

If you notice that when you stop drinking, you experience withdrawal symptoms, you need to be medically detoxified, as it can be dangerous for you to stop drinking on your own. During medical detoxification, you will be monitored and given medication to offset any withdrawal symptoms so that, gradually and safely, your body will get used to no longer having alcohol. Even if you do not experience a withdrawal syndrome when you stop drinking, it is a good idea to get checked out by your physician. Heavy drinking can cause other medical problems, and your doctor can ensure that you are healthy and do not have any serious health concerns. While detoxification usually takes place on an inpatient basis, if your withdrawal syndrome is not too severe, you may be able to be detoxified as an outpatient with physician oversight.

Detoxification, however, is only the first step. Learning how to stop alcohol from ruining your life is the next objective.

CHAPTER 7

What to Do: Abstinence or Moderation?

People are usually more convinced by reasons they discovered
themselves than by those found by others.
BLAISE PASCAL

Okay, you are now ready to stop alcohol from hurting your life. In order to do this, you need to change your relationship with alcohol. You are probably wondering whether you should try to moderate your drinking or whether you need to stop drinking entirely.

As a first choice, many, if not most, people prefer to control alcohol intake so that it stops causing problems in their life. At least at some point, most people who drink too much have entertained this desire. They want to continue to drink and have that pleasure but without all of the problems that formerly went with it. They want to be like other people who drink safely and without doing themselves or others harm. Non-problem drinkers seldom, if ever, drink to excess; they generally do not become seriously intoxicated; and overall, alcohol does not interfere in their life. Simply put, no problems result from their moderate alcohol consumption. The way to end your problems may be to learn how to drink in moderation.

On the other hand, there are others who may know already that trying to control their drinking is simply not possible. They have tried to limit the amount they drink numerous times, and inevitably their drinking got out of control again. For such people, the goal is to learn how to achieve abstinence from alcohol because they know from experience that this will be the only path to success.

There may be yet other people, though, who truly do not know what they should do. Their alcohol use has become problematic, but they are not sure what's the best path to take. This chapter will help you make that decision.

TRYING TO MODERATE DRINKING IS CONTROVERSIAL

As I discussed in chapter 2, many people and professional organizations maintain that a drinking problem is a disease and that the best, if not only, way to recover from a drinking problem is by abstaining from alcohol. Alcoholics Anonymous, for one, believes that abstinence is the only way to recover from a drinking problem. Remember, from the point of view that an alcohol problem is a disease, any drinking will eventually escalate to overdrinking because the "loss of control" phenomenon is part of the illness. In this view, alcoholics find it simply impossible to moderate their drinking permanently, and in truth, many people who drink too much can't control their drinking. One drink leads to way too many.

Yet Some People Can Do It

As I also discussed in chapter 2, in contrast to the disease perspective, a drinking problem can be considered a bad habit. This perspective opens the door to the possibility that a person can learn to drink differently. I mentioned that an alcohol use disorder runs along a continuum of severity. Some individuals have a severe form of the disorder, whereas others have a milder case. In fact, many people who have experienced a problem with alcohol have learned to change their destructive pattern of drinking. So, although the technique of moderating drinking is controversial, it is clearly possible for some people to do it.

How Common Is Moderate Drinking?

Reports of individuals learning how to control their drinking after having had a problem with drinking vary from study to study. Some studies report that only about 5 percent of people who have experienced a drinking problem can learn to moderate their drinking. Not very good odds. Yet other studies report that 30 percent or even 60 percent of people who have had a drinking problem can learn moderation. Obviously, much better odds. Why the huge range?

My own practice mirrors these findings. I sometimes find that three or even four out of five people who want to control their drinking are able to. But at another time, I might find that only one out of five can do this, or maybe no one can. Again, why the range and what is responsible for this? Variation in the rates of successful moderation reported in studies is due to several factors, including how long ago people first experienced an alcohol problem, how controlled drinking is defined, and, most important, who is actually studied.

In general, the longer ago people first experienced an alcohol problem, the more likely they are to report controlling their drinking. The same is true for abstinence-oriented outcomes because, over time, people with alcohol problems get better either by abstaining or by learning to moderate their drinking. By contrast, for people who report that they recently experienced a problem with alcohol, the percentage who are moderating their drinking is less, which is also true for rates of abstinence. Again, over time, people get better, whether they learn to moderate their drinking or instead decide to abstain. How controlled drinking is defined in these studies is also important. Obviously, with a strict definition of controlled drinking, there will be fewer reports of success, whereas with a more liberal definition, the number of people who manage to moderate their drinking will be greater.

Finally, and most important, is the severity of drinker being studied, which can greatly affect the observed rates of successful controlled drinking. Individuals with a more severe alcohol problem seem to do best with an abstinence approach, whereas those with a less severe problem are better able to learn how to moderate their drinking.

Related to the severity of the alcohol problem is the fact that rates of controlled drinking are also greater for individuals who never received treatment for their alcohol problem. In general, people who seek treatment for a drinking problem have more significant troubles with alcohol than those who have not received treatment. Typically, an alcohol problem goes on for many years before a person is willing to get involved in treatment. A person often avoids treatment until there is outside pressure to seek it, and often the pressure results from consistent and severe problems related to alcohol consumption. As a result, if a study looks only at people who received treatment, the rates of controlled drinking are lower. Furthermore, because most treatment programs focus exclusively on abstinence as the only route to recovery, those who have received treatment are more likely to choose the abstinence path to resolve their problem as opposed to individuals who have helped themselves without treatment. In turn, rates of controlled drinking among individuals who have received treatment will be lower.

It Depends on the Person

The truth of the matter is that there is such variation in the findings because the outcome depends on who the person is and the type of drinking problem he or she has. Drinking problems vary in type and severity, so some people have a higher probability of learning how to moderate their drinking, whereas others have a smaller chance. So what are your chances of learning to moderate your drinking?

Who Can Moderate Their Drinking?

You'll have the best chance of learning how to moderate your drinking if these conditions apply to you:

- You have never been physically dependent on alcohol (have never experienced the alcohol withdrawal syndrome described in chapter 6).

- You are not a daily drinker.

- You have had a drinking problem for less than 10 years. Think about your history of drinking. You may have started drinking a long time ago, but have you had a drinking *problem* for a long time? If you have, your chances of successfully moderating your drinking are less.

- You have not had severe problems related to drinking. Think long and hard about the effect alcohol has had on your life. Has drinking caused you severe problems like losing jobs and relationships, having legal troubles, or suffering other major hardships?

- You have had past periods of successfully not drinking or of moderating your drinking.

- You are employed. Employment structures your day and improves your chances of successful moderate drinking.

- You are psychologically stable. Is drinking your main problem, or do you struggle with other emotional concerns such as significant depression or anxiety?

- You have friends and family who are not heavy drinkers.

- You are under age 40. (Age matters because it correlates with the number of years of drinking.)

- You very much want to moderate your drinking.

- You have a social environment that supports moderate drinking. Not only is it important that the people around you aren't heavy drinkers, but you also need people around you who support your wish to moderate your drinking.

Before you try this approach, and if you are taking any prescribed medication, you should check with your doctor first to see if you can drink while taking your medication. And if you are pregnant, you should not drink alcohol at all, as it can have harmful effects on your fetus. A good recommendation before attempting controlled drinking is to get a physical exam from your doctor to confirm that drinking will not cause a medical problem for you.

WHO SHOULD CHOOSE ABSTINENCE?

You'll do best with an abstinence approach if the following conditions apply to you:

- You have had a drinking problem for more than 10 years. Take a good look at your drinking history and the effect that alcohol has had on your life. If your misuse of alcohol has been going on for many years, you'll do best by stopping drinking entirely.

- You drink every day or rarely have days when you don't drink.

- You have experienced many problems from your drinking. Again, take a long and hard look at the influence alcohol has had on your life. Has it caused you many problems, whether in lost jobs, broken relationships, legal difficulties, or financial struggles?

- You have had periods of heavy drinking, and during those times, you have been unable to function and keep up your daily activities.

- You have been or are physically dependent on alcohol. When you stop drinking, do you experience the alcohol withdrawal syndrome described in chapter 6?

- You have been told by your doctor not to drink.

- You have a medical condition that could be worsened by drinking.

- You are pregnant or trying to become pregnant.

- You have previously tried to moderate your drinking with only limited success because each time your drinking got out of control again.

- You are surrounded by heavy drinkers. If your social network of friends and family includes heavy drinkers, chances are that you will need to abstain from alcohol to prevent it from hurting your life.

Many people intuitively know whether they will need to abstain from alcohol to recover from their alcohol problem. From their history, they know that, for themselves, one drink inevitably leads to too many and that total abstinence will be the only way to avoid this. They may have tried numerous times to control their drinking without success. If this sounds familiar to you, I would suggest the route of abstinence.

ABSTINENCE OR MODERATION?

Perhaps you've read my recommendations, and even though you don't fit the description of someone who is likely to be able to control drinking through moderation, you still want to try to learn how to control it. You think that, with effort, you may be able to achieve success. Who knows, you *may* be right. There are people who have had severe problems with alcohol who, much to my surprise, beat the odds. I can only speak of tendencies and probabilities, which might not account for individual variation.

This book is about your taking control of how you want to address your problem with alcohol. Even if the chances are against your being able to learn to drink in moderation, you may still want to try. You may feel that you first need to see whether you can do this before you consider abstinence. If this is what you want to do, go for it. However, again, if this is your plan, first check with your doctor to make sure that it is okay for you to drink at all.

ONE CAVEAT

Some of you may have resolved your alcohol problem by not drinking at all. If abstinence is working for you, don't change a thing. As the saying goes, "If it's not broken, don't fix it." Stay the course if it's working.

SUMMARY

In this chapter, I explained what type of drinker has the best chance of resolving a drinking problem by learning how to drink moderately and what type should choose the path of abstinence. Now is the time for you to decide which category you fit into. Reread the bullet-list profiles and take an honest look at yourself and your relationship to alcohol. Decide which category best describes you, and commit to a course of action. Now is the time to stop alcohol from ruining your life and to start feeling better about yourself. No matter what your decision, the very fact that you recognize you have a problem is something to be proud of.

The next part of this book is devoted to strategies to help you moderate your drinking. If your decision is to abstain, skip to part IV. Either of these paths can help; you just need to follow the correct one for you. Good luck—but know that it takes more than luck. It takes a commitment to change your life and to hard work. If you keep this in mind, you will succeed.

PART III

Moderating
Your Drinking

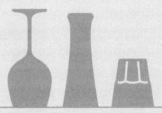

CHAPTER 8

Moderation:
General Techniques

To enjoy freedom we have to control ourselves.
VIRGINIA WOOLF

Moderation means being able to control and limit your drinking to a level that does not interfere with your life. Your goal is to learn to drink in a way that does not cause you financial, vocational, physical, legal, emotional, or social difficulties. To accomplish this, the amount of alcohol you consume must stay within a reasonable limit and be less than what you used to drink. There are many techniques to help you moderate your drinking. These techniques must be the practices behind the individualized moderate drinking contract you will develop in the next chapter.

SIP AND ENJOY YOUR DRINKS

Sipping your drinks will greatly slow down your drinking and make it easier for you to moderate your alcohol intake. Try putting your drink on the table or bar between sips. This will slow you down because continuing to hold your drink leads to more rapid drinking. If the drink remains in your hand, it's too easy to drink it quickly. You'll be surprised at how long you can make a drink last and how much you will still enjoy drinking. One way to make this transition easier is to play a game with yourself to see how slowly you can finish a drink.

See if you can make your drink last for one hour, or if that seems too long, at least 45 minutes.

Another suggestion is to focus on the flavor of the drink. Typically, people who drink too much chug their drinks and don't even taste what they are drinking. They drink to get drunk, which is exactly what you do not want to do. You need to focus on the taste rather than on getting drunk.

TAKE A BREAK BETWEEN DRINKS

Try taking a break between your drinks. So often, as soon as one drink is finished, a person may immediately, without really thinking, have another one. Instead, take some time between drinks, which will slow down your drinking. Another technique is to have a nonalcoholic drink in between alcoholic ones. Again, this will greatly slow down your drinking and will make controlling your use of alcohol much easier. While you may not do this in between every alcoholic drink, you can do it at least some of the time.

DON'T DRINK SHOTS, MULTI-SHOT DRINKS, OR PUNCHES

In light of what I just said, it makes sense that you should stay away from drinking shots of hard liquor because it is hard to make a shot last a long time. Drinking shots is an easy way to drink too quickly and too much.

You should also stay away from multi-shot drinks such as a mai tai, Long Island Iced Tea, or Black Russian. These have more alcohol content in them than single-shot mixed drinks and do not qualify as just *one* drink. They are much stronger and tend to be drunk too quickly as well.

Punches are also dangerous because you don't always know what type of alcohol is in them or how strong they are. You may think that you are having only one drink, but in reality the alcohol content may equal two or more drinks. They are also easy to gulp down, especially if you're thirsty.

MEASURE YOUR DRINK

I recommend, at least when you are first trying to control your drinking, to measure your drinks. A standard drink is about 12 ounces of beer, which is usually about 4–5 percent alcohol; 5 ounces of wine, which is about 12 percent alcohol; or 1.5 ounces of distilled spirits, which is about 40 percent alcohol, or 80 proof. I would use these guidelines when measuring your drinks. When you do this, you may be surprised at the smaller amount of alcohol in a standard drink compared with the ones you were used to drinking.

You should also know that many beers are now much stronger than 4–5 percent alcohol. Many new craft beers have 6–8 percent alcohol, and some can even approach 12–14 percent. When you develop your individualized moderate drinking contract in the next chapter, which will include how much you should drink, these potencies are important to keep in mind.

Remember, too, when drinking at a bar, that so often the drinks served are larger than standard drinks. A gin and tonic or vodka cocktail poured by a bartender may contain two to three times the amount of alcohol as a standard drink. Beers served in glasses can also be much more than 12 ounces, and wine pours can be quite generous as well. Especially when you are first trying to control your drinking, ensure that you stick to standard drinks.

To drive this point home, get a martini glass and put 1.5 ounces of water in it and see how little this is. Add another 3 ounces, which is now equivalent to three standard drinks, and this is probably closer to the size of a martini you might get served at a bar. Again, be honest with yourself and stick to standard drinks.

DON'T DRINK WHEN YOU'RE THIRSTY

When people are thirsty, they drink fluid to relieve their thirst. If you drink alcohol when you are thirsty, you will tend to drink more quickly and in all probability will drink more. Alcohol can actually make you thirstier because it dehydrates you. Drinking alcohol causes you to sweat, increases the production of urine, and results in a loss of body water. So when you drink alcohol to quench your thirst, it has the opposite effect. When you are thirsty, the best thing to drink is water. Have a glass or two of water first to quench your thirst before drinking any alcohol.

EAT WHEN YOU DRINK

Eat when you drink, and never drink on an empty stomach. Having food in your stomach will slow down the rate at which alcohol gets into your bloodstream. This will help diminish the effects of alcohol and will prevent the rapid intoxication that can lead you to make poorer decisions about your drinking. Some people I have worked with reported that when they are full after eating, their desire to drink is greatly lessened. As a result, eating before drinking has helped them decrease their alcohol consumption. One note of caution, though, when eating and drinking: don't eat salty foods, which increase your thirst and lead to more drinking. Stay away from peanuts, chips, fries, and other salty snacks.

KEEP A LIMITED SUPPLY OF ALCOHOL AT HOME

If you drink mostly when you are at home, you shouldn't keep a lot of alcohol on hand. Having alcohol readily accessible can make drinking, and overdrinking, way too tempting. Limiting the amount of alcohol you keep around your home will help you moderate your drinking.

PREPARE YOUR MINDSET

When you plan to drink or know that you will be in a drinking situation, you must remind yourself that you are trying to limit your drinking. You need to prepare yourself in advance and enter these situations with a focused and determined mindset. You must remind yourself that you are no longer drinking to get drunk, which is out of the question. Rather, you are drinking to enjoy the taste of alcohol and to enjoy the social situation you are in.

In the next chapter, you will learn how to create your individualized moderate drinking contract, which will help ensure that your drinking stays within safe limits. Once you have developed your contract, think about it and be determined to follow it before entering any social situation.

DELAY HAVING YOUR FIRST ALCOHOLIC DRINK

When you first enter a drinking situation, wait to have your first alcoholic drink. Give yourself time to adjust to and enjoy the setting without using alcohol. After you are already enjoying yourself, have a drink if you want. Waiting a while will help get you in the right frame of mind—the one in which you keep a watchful eye on your drinking. If you really need to have a drink in your hand to feel at ease, make it one without alcohol.

In a similar vein, if your pattern has been to have a drink when you first get home from work, wait to have that drink. Have something nonalcoholic if you need something to drink, or simply wait to have that initial drink. You can even disrupt your usual pattern by doing something before going home, like running an errand or going to the gym. Delaying that initial drink will help slow down your drinking.

STAY FOCUSED ON MODERATION

In a social situation where everyone is drinking, you need to stay focused and not allow yourself to get caught up in the camaraderie of heavy drinking. For example, when a group of people are out to dinner and one in the group orders another drink, frequently everyone else at the table follows suit without thinking too much about whether they really want another. Or, if a person is buying a drink for himself, he may offer to buy drinks for others; again, without thinking much about it, everyone jumps on the bandwagon. You need to be mindful of these scenarios.

GET PLEASURE FROM THE SOCIAL SITUATION

When in a social situation, even though drinking may be a part of the scene, there is much more to do than drink. You can meet new people, reconnect with old friends, or listen to music. Whether you are playing softball, swimming, dancing, or playing cards, you can keep the focus on controlling your drinking while getting your enjoyment from everything else going on around you. If you can center your energy on all the other pleasurable aspects of the situation, you'll naturally put less emphasis on drinking. You may find that you enjoy these things more now that you are concentrating less on getting drunk.

LET'S GET STARTED

The best way to begin your new life of moderation is to take a one-month break from drinking before you start to try to control your drinking. If that sounds too long, try to go two weeks without alcohol, or at least one week, although I recommend two. This break from alcohol is helpful for a number of reasons.

First, with moderate drinking, I strongly recommend that you do not drink every day. I know this can be a challenge if you are used to drinking most every day. But relax; you can do this. You may find that while it is initially somewhat challenging not to drink, within a fairly short period of time, it gets much easier. You will get used to not drinking, and taking a one-month or two-week break will boost your confidence in your ability not to drink. This will be very useful once you actually start your plan to moderate your drinking.

Second, for many of you, moderate drinking will be a lifestyle change. You will be drinking less, and less often, than you presently do, and you may need to find other things to do with your time. During this fairly brief period of not drinking, experiment with a new hobby or spend more time on one you have always enjoyed. Filling your time with rewarding activities will be valuable in keeping alcohol from being a major part of your life forever. Get used to what it feels like not to drink, which will be useful self-knowledge once you implement your moderate drinking contract.

There may be certain times when you miss drinking or when you feel like drinking more than at other times. Again, not drinking will build your confidence and let you know that, despite wanting to drink, you can choose not to. Also, discovering when you really want to drink can give you insight into the role that alcohol plays in your life and what you need to manage without it. For example, if you feel like drinking after a stressful day at work, you will need to find other ways to relax after a long day. Or if you feel like drinking more when you are angry or upset, you can work on learning to cope with these feelings in other ways.

MODERATING YOUR DRINKING
ISN'T SOCIAL DRINKING

A social drinker does not think about when to drink, how to drink, how much to drink, or what type of alcohol to drink. A social drinker does not need to prepare her mindset and doesn't worry about getting drunk or the possibility that drinking can get out of control and cause problems. For social drinkers, alcohol is simply not an issue: they can take it or leave it.

For someone who is moderating his drinking, though, drinking is an issue that needs to be taken seriously. Moderate drinkers must *always* remain vigilant and mindful of how much they drink because the possibility of drinking too much remains all too real. They must also remember all of the mental attitudes that will enable them to succeed at moderate drinking: committing decisively to change, admitting the harmful consequences of excessive alcohol consumption, affirming the vision you have for yourself and what you want your life to be, finding joy in life without drinking and not wanting to lose that, and being able to deal with life stress and internal urges without turning to alcohol.

SUMMARY

In this chapter, I reviewed general techniques for you to use that will help you moderate your drinking. These methods will likely change the way you have been drinking. They are what you need to practice in order to stop alcohol from causing you problems. The following should become "standard operating procedures" that govern your drinking:

- Sip, slow down, and enjoy your drinks.
- Take a break between drinks.
- Avoid shots, multi-shot drinks, and punches.
- Measure your drinks, at least initially, and notice the portions served to you at bars and restaurants.
- Don't drink alcoholic beverages when you are thirsty.
- Eat when you drink.

• Have a limited supply of alcohol at home.

• Whenever you drink, prepare your mindset by keeping moderation in your thoughts and remembering to stay focused on your reasons for choosing to drink less.

• Delay having your first alcoholic drink.

• When you are in a drinking situation, remain vigilant and mindful of moderation.

• Enjoy the situation you are in; alcohol should only be a small part of it.

Let's now turn in chapter 9 to the elements of the moderate drinking contract you will develop and learn to live by.

CHAPTER 9

Your Personal Moderate Drinking Contract

*Unless commitment is made, there are only
promises and hopes; but no plans.*
PETER F. DRUCKER

To learn to moderate your drinking and to make it as easy as possible, you need to make a contract with yourself that clearly outlines how much, how often, and when and where you can drink. You can't simply "cut down" or make a conscious decision to drink less. This contract with yourself symbolizes your *total commitment to yourself* to get your drinking under control and specifies clear rules for you to drink and live by.

WHY ARE CLEAR RULES IMPORTANT?

Rules give you structure, which is essential because your drinking has been out of control. Laying out clear drinking rules gives you the firm guidelines you need to bring your drinking under control. Safe drinking rules that you agree to follow provide explicit targets and goals and a clear path to pursue to limit your drinking. Without such rules, chances are you won't get a handle on your drinking.

Developing rules that you decide to follow is also a good way for you to know whether or not you can truly moderate your drinking—*not some of the time but all of the time.* If you cannot abide by the rules you set for your moderate drinking, that means you can't moderate your drinking and that abstinence is the better route for you.

Setting rules will prevent you from slipping back into old habits. For example, let's assume that you used to drink two six-packs of beer and have decided to cut down, without prescribing rules. In cutting down, some days you drink four beers, other days you drink six, and over time, your drinking increases so that sometimes you drink eight or ten. While you have cut down, is this truly moderating your drinking? Clearly not. Developing precise limits on how much you can and will safely drink—*all of the time*—will keep you on track and prevent your drinking from escalating.

THE SEVEN CRUCIAL QUESTIONS OF YOUR MODERATE DRINKING CONTRACT

In this chapter, you'll learn the specific elements of your moderate drinking contract by answering seven crucial questions. Before you fill out the contract that appears near the end of this chapter, you have to understand each of these elements that will allow you to succeed. This contract will be the document you will live by as you learn to moderate your drinking. You will also be asked to think about things that you will do to support this lifestyle change. But first, the seven key questions.

1. How Much Can You Drink?

The first question you need to answer is how many drinks you can safely consume in one sitting. I believe that a maximum of three standard drinks is more than enough for any person. Three drinks is the upper limit because this amount is not enough to intoxicate most people. (Of course, if you become intoxicated by three drinks, your personal limit should be lower.) When you drink more than this amount, your judgment can become impaired, making it difficult to exercise good decision-making. Adhering to this limit is crucial to complying with your drinking contract. At the beginning, you may even want to consider limiting yourself to a maximum of two drinks. You want to succeed, and the more conservative number of two drinks may ensure that your drinking does not escalate, as committing to having only two drinks puts even more focus on limiting your alcohol consumption.

If you are struggling with the two- or three-drink limit, you may increase your limit to four, but I don't recommend this when you start off. Later on, after you have demonstrated good control, it may be possible for you to be somewhat more flexible with this limit. For now, though, stick to a three-drink limit. If you can't be satisfied with three drinks, moderate drinking may not be the right option for you.

When suggesting drinking limits, you should know that the National Institute on Alcohol Abuse and Alcoholism suggests that women drink no more than 1 drink per day or 7 drinks per week and that men should consume a maximum of 2 drinks per day or 14 drinks per week. The World Health Organization has a somewhat more liberal recommendation for low-risk drinking: about 3 drinks per day or 21 drinks per week for men and slightly less than 2 drinks per day or about 14 drinks per week for women. Men who drink 5 or more drinks in a day or more than 15 in a week, and women who drink 4 or more in a day or 8 in a week, have an increased risk of developing alcohol-related problems.

These are general guidelines, and everyone is different. A person's metabolism, age, weight, and medical status all affect how alcohol interacts with that person's body. So I strongly recommend that you speak with your physician about what your limit should be when deciding how many drinks you can have in one sitting.

As I just mentioned, weight is a factor, as heavier people generally can handle more alcohol than those who weigh less. So when thinking about your limit, take this into account, and if you weigh less than the average woman or man, go with a lower limit.

You should also know that, for some people, four drinks or even three may be too many because this can easily turn into drinking five or six. If this is the case for you, limit yourself to a maximum of one or two.

What Is a Drink? When setting guidelines for the number of drinks you can have, we need to talk about what counts as *a drink*. A standard drink is equivalent to a 12-ounce bottle of beer, five ounces of wine, or one-and-a-half ounces of 80-proof hard liquor. These are "honest," measured drinks and not the tumbler-size ones you may have occasionally consumed. When pouring drinks, you will need to start measuring them, at least initially. Once you get used to these amounts, you may be able to gauge them without measuring. But no cheating, as you will only be kidding yourself.

As I mentioned in the last chapter, the alcohol content of beer can vary greatly, from 4–5 percent to as high as 12–14 percent. When deciding how many drinks you can have when it is beer, one drink of beer should have an alcohol content in the 4–5 percent range and not be stronger. Or if you choose a stronger beer, take that into account, as one of those could well count as two drinks.

Women Are Different from Men. As I just noted, recommendations from leading health agencies for low-risk drinking set lower limits for women than for men. Women have a higher proportion of fat in their bodies in relation to water and tend to feel the effects of alcohol more than men do. This is why I agree with the guidelines that set lower limits for women. For women, keeping to a three-drink limit, or even two, is strongly recommended because of physiology.

You Can Drink Less but Never More! Just because your upper limit is three doesn't mean you must *always* drink that many. In fact, a good sign of being able to control your drinking is that you can choose to have only one or two on some days. This doesn't mean, however, that you can go over your limit on other days.

Slow Down, and Don't Gulp Your Drinks. Consume only one drink per hour or at least make your drink last close to one hour. This prevents intoxication and will decrease the chances of your having alcohol-related problems. Looking at a clock and pacing your drinking is critical to your success. Sipping your drink, putting your drink down, and focusing on the taste will help you to do this. (Review the practices described in chapter 8.)

Don't Forget about Nonalcoholic Drinks. It is useful to intersperse nonalcoholic drinks with alcoholic ones, especially in social situations where you are used to having a drink in your hands. Nonalcoholic drinks include water or sparkling water, soda, fruit juice, or even nonalcoholic beer or wine. There is certainly nothing wrong with holding and drinking any one of these nonalcoholic drinks. Have as many as you like. Drinking in this fashion will help keep your alcohol consumption in control.

Start Off with a Nonalcoholic Drink. Particularly when in social situations, start off with a nonalcoholic drink. Your mindset is key (see chapter 8). If you know that you are going to be somewhere for a long time and drinking is a part of the scene, starting with an alcohol-free beverage will help you focus on limiting your drinking and keeping it in control. Your mindset will be on moderating your drinking and not on getting drunk.

For example, Kathy usually drank without any problems, except on the weekends when socializing and drinking with a group of friends. In that setting, she would often overdrink, which was beginning to cause problems between her and her husband. She also didn't like how she felt the next day. Her trick to limiting her intake was to begin the evening with one or two nonalcoholic drinks, which would delay the start of her drinking. She learned that doing this set the stage for her entire evening: instead of jumping into the evening with alcohol to feel its effects, this delay kept her focused on moderating her drinking, and she enjoyed the evening while having only two or three alcoholic drinks.

Make Sure to Eat. Not only is it a good idea to eat food when you drink; it's an even better idea to eat something *before* drinking. Having food in your stomach slows the rate at which alcohol enters your system. This, in turn, decreases the effect alcohol has on you and makes it easier to adhere to your drinking limit.

2. What Can You Drink?

While typically "a drink is a drink is a drink," and all alcoholic drinks have the capacity to cause you to lose control, it is possible that a certain kind of alcohol may cause you more of a problem than others. For example, some people can drink beer without a problem, but if they drink hard liquor, even when diluted, it's another story. Others find they can maintain control by sticking to wine. In fact, unless diluted, hard liquor, with its greater percentage of alcohol, gets into your system more quickly than does a drink with a lower percentage of alcohol such as beer or wine. So, remember, it is harder to maintain control if you drink hard liquor. Limiting alcohol consumption to only beer or wine will help you maintain control.

Just as you can alternate alcoholic beverages with nonalcoholic ones to help limit your drinking, if you still want to be able to drink hard liquor, it may work for you to dilute your hard liquor with a greater amount of mixer. Drinking this way helps make a drink last much longer and will help keep your drinking in control.

Switching to a less preferred alcoholic beverage can also help you control drinking. For example, if wine is your favorite beverage and what you always drink, changing to beer can help you drink less.

If you are an individual who runs into problems no matter what you drink, or you start off with a less preferred beverage but soon go back to your favorite, problematic one, you need to remain abstinent to resolve your drinking problem. For you, "a drink is a drink is a drink."

3. How Often Can You Drink?
A good guideline is to drink three or at most four days per week. Of course, drinking less is always a good choice.

The Four-Day Limit. Drinking more than four days per week is dangerous because frequent drinking can escalate to daily drinking, which increases the chances of repeating your alcohol-related problems. If you can't imagine having some days on which you do not drink, then moderate drinking is not for you and you should choose total abstinence.

Going three days every week without alcohol lessens the likelihood you'll develop a tolerance to alcohol. Tolerance is when your body gets used to alcohol and you need more of it to feel an effect.

Remember back when one drink used to make you feel relaxed? Over time, you probably needed two drinks to create the same feeling, then three or even four. Abstinent days are important in helping you moderate your drinking. Maybe you can think about drinking on the weekends but limiting your drinking during the week.

Having days without drinking forces you to do other things with your life that do not include or revolve around drinking. This is key, since moderate drinking demands that you change your lifestyle. Having other activities you enjoy doing makes moderating your drinking much easier. For example, instead of your usual pattern of going home after work and drinking, go to the health club, go shopping, see a movie, enroll in a class, or meet some friends for coffee. Or if you go home, change your usual routine and take a walk or jog, read a book, involve yourself in a house project, or develop some other leisure activity.

Nondrinking days also break the habit of daily drinking, which in and of itself can be helpful for moderating your drinking. It forces you to get used to doing things other than drinking, which, over time, will become your routine. Not drinking some days will eventually become your "new normal."

4. When Can You Drink . . . and 5. When Can't You Drink?

Your next step is to establish the types of situations in which you can drink and, equally as important, the types of situations in which you should avoid drinking. Over the course of your life, you, like everyone who drinks, has developed a drinking pattern. There are times or situations when your drinking is generally in control and you only have a few drinks. There are also times when your drinking becomes excessive. If you are going to control your drinking consistently, you need to analyze your drinking pattern to pinpoint your "low risk" and "high risk" situations.

Low risk means those situations you are in, or people you are with, where you have been able to drink safely. *High risk* means the places, times, or people that cause you to drink too much. You need to identify those situations that are low risk for you and make a rule to drink only in those situations. You also need to identify your high-risk situations and make a rule never to drink when in them.

For example, Al, a successful 38-year-old father of two children, discovered that he would never overdrink when he drank at home with his family around. However, when he stopped off at the local tavern after work with some of his coworkers, he would generally drink too much and arrive home late, and problems would ensue between him and his wife. One of his rules was to drink only when at home with his family and never to drink at the tavern.

Charlie, 29 years old and single, realized that with certain friends who were not heavy drinkers, he would never lose control of his drinking. However, with another group, his friends from high school who drank heavily, he would often drink too much. To moderate his drinking, he made a rule not to drink with his high school friends and to see them less often.

Times of the Day. There may be particular times during your daily routine when you tend to slip in a drink or two, which then often leads to more. If there are, make the rule not to drink during those times. Mary, a 32-year-old married woman, realized that if she began to drink while preparing dinner for her family, she would often drink too much. However, if she waited until she sat down with her family for dinner to have her first drink, she would not overdrink, and her drinking was much easier to control. Bob discovered that if he first started to drink at home before going out to a bar, he would drink too much. However, if he waited to have his first drink at the bar, he could control his drinking. Finally, Andy, a 69-year-old retired married man, discovered that when he began to drink around two o'clock in the afternoon, he generally would overdrink and be a little too intoxicated when his wife returned home from work at half past five o'clock. He learned that he had a much easier time controlling his drinking if he waited to have his first drink about four o'clock, and he made it his rule never to drink before that time.

On the flip side, there are people who tend to drink too long and too late after they begin to drink. This leads to too much drinking. For them, a good rule would be never to drink past a certain hour in the evening. Tom, a 55-year-old married man, realized that he would typically extend his drinking after dinner, which resulted in his drinking much more than he wanted. He decided to make a rule that he would no longer drink after finishing his dinner. Elizabeth, a 32-year-old single woman, found that when out with her friends, she would continue to drink until late into the evening, which resulted in her getting too intoxicated. She made a hard and fast rule never to order a drink past ten o'clock, which helped her remain in control.

Your State of Mind. While a person can always find a reason to drink, there may be certain psychological states that tend to trigger your heavier drinking. For example, painful emotional states—anger, loneliness, sadness, stress, or frustration—are often triggers.

Think about whether there are feelings that have historically spurred your drinking. What are they? Once you list them, make the decision not to drink when feeling that way. Obviously, you will need to develop other ways to manage your feelings, especially the painful ones. You should think of more constructive things to do and healthier ways to cope when you are feeling bad. Talking with a friend, taking a warm bath, going for a jog, listening to music, reading a book, or meditating are just a few examples of other things you can do to cope with difficult feelings.

For example, Wayne noticed that whenever he had a stressful day at work, he liked to relax with a drink before having dinner with his wife. During these times, he often lost control of his drinking. As a way to moderate his alcohol intake, he made a rule never to drink during these times of stress. Instead, he learned other ways to relax, which included meditation, reading, and exercise. He also was surprised to find that sitting down with his wife before dinner with only a club soda and lemon helped him unwind as well. It was taking the time to relax and talk about his day, rather than the alcohol per se, that did the trick.

6. What Situations Should You Totally Avoid?

Despite your best intentions not to drink when in any of your high-risk situations, you may find that this is simply not possible. For example, most of your friends may be heavy drinkers. You may have decided not to drink when you're with these friends because your drinking is heavier when you're around them. Even if you resolve not to drink in this situation, in truth it may be very difficult if not impossible. A better rule for you would be not to put yourself in such a situation in the first place.

Several years ago, I worked with Sam, a 43-year-old married man who wanted to learn to control his drinking. In reviewing his drinking with me, Sam realized that whenever he went out to dinner with his wife, he could consistently have one or two drinks and would never overdrink. However, whenever he socialized with a particular set of heavy-drinking friends in group settings, he would regularly drink too much, although he had made a rule never to drink when he saw these friends. He discovered that whenever he socialized with them, he couldn't refrain from drinking (and from drinking too much). He was forced to make a rule to stop seeing these friends in group situations. Fortunately, Sam didn't have to give up these friends entirely. He spoke with them and was able to see them on an individual basis when heavy drinking was not in the picture. He also found that if he went out to dinner with his wife, and one of his friends and his friend's wife joined them, he could moderate his drinking as well.

Tom was a 23-year-old single man who came to me at his lawyer's suggestion. While extremely intoxicated, he had been arrested for breaking into a retail store. Although he didn't remember why he had broken into the store, he had a vague recollection of the police finding him in the store after he set off the burglar alarm. Tom was a heavy drinker who would stop off at a bar a couple of times each week and could consume between one and two quarts of gin when he drank. He rarely drank at home and realized that the only time he drank so heavily was when he met his friends at the bar. As a way to control his drinking, he decided that he could only drink at home and never go to the bar, where he knew he would overdrink.

7. What Other Activities Will You Start to Do?

Drinking too much can interfere with your life by taking the focus off other things in your life that are important to you. Some examples might include no longer working out or engaging in physical activity, being less attentive to and engaged with a family member, letting house projects go unfinished, not being involved in other leisure activities, or having allowed some leisure activities you used to do slip away. Or perhaps there is something you want to accomplish, but drinking has obstructed that.

Along with making rules that govern your drinking, you should think about and write down activities or interests that you will begin to pursue. These do not need to be great and noble causes, although they could be, because even small things can support and make you feel good about your lifestyle change. Consider, too, how your drinking may have affected your overall life and others around you, and reflect on whether there are some changes you should make.

For example, Anthony admitted that most of the childcare responsibilities on weekend mornings fell to his wife because he had been drinking too much the night before. He committed to helping her, which his wife greatly appreciated, and he enjoyed being more involved with his children. Elizabeth had a bicycle that she no longer used since drinking had become her mainstay activity after work. She committed to riding again as a part of her commitment to change her life. Rebecca had always wanted to get involved in a wildlife conservation organization but had never got around to it. As a part of her plan, she researched and decided to join a local conservation group. Doing these things not only gives you other things to do with your time, which can make controlling drinking easier, but your involvement also will add value to your life and help you appreciate the benefits of getting your drinking under control.

THREE IMPORTANT CONTRACT RULES

So now you understand the seven questions to answer for your moderate drinking contract. Before you get started on writing your contract, however, there are three other rules you need to know.

1. Don't Be Discouraged

Don't be discouraged if your spouse or other family members or your drinking buddies think that your goal of trying to moderate your drinking is ridiculous. They probably have good reason to think so. How often have they heard you say, "I won't drink that much, just a couple," only to watch you proceed to overdrink? Or perhaps you stopped drinking for some time and then started again, leading to your drinking eventually getting out of control.

You need to remember that most people, including your family members, believe that abstinence is the only way to resolve a drinking problem. They may think that trying to moderate your drinking is simply a fantasy born of your unwillingness to admit you have a problem. As a result, family members may think that the whole idea of you trying to moderate your drinking is doomed to fail. They may feel angry that you are continuing to drink, or at a minimum, they will be confused about what you are doing. The key is not to be discouraged if you firmly believe you are able to moderate your drinking.

Getting Support for a Moderate Drinking Contract. Communicate, communicate, and communicate. Talk with your spouse, family members, or others close to you who have been affected by your drinking. Talk about what you are doing, and after you complete your moderate drinking contract, show it to them and try to enlist their support. Make sure they understand what you are attempting to do so that you will have their backing. Explain to them that their support will help you more than their confusion, resentment, or anger.

Don't simply say to them that you are trying to "cut down" your drinking. How many times have you probably said this to them already? Rather, explain to them that you are trying to moderate your drinking and show them your moderate drinking contract. This will demonstrate how well you have thought this out. You should also let them know that you plan to stop drinking entirely if you can't successfully moderate your drinking. This should ease their concern about what you are attempting to do and help you gain their support.

I am reminded of Steve, a 46-year-old successful businessman who had been married to Sandy for 14 years. Prior to seeing me, Steve had just been discharged from an inpatient detoxification program after being referred there by his employer. For the previous three years, Steve had been drinking at least five times per week and had consumed one or two pints of gin each night. Steve used to smoke marijuana daily, and when his supply ran out, he turned to alcohol. Steve drank at home after work to relieve tension, and his drinking had greatly affected his relationship with his wife. In fact, Steve and Sandy were sleeping in separate bedrooms, and she was considering a separation. Both of Steve's parents were alcoholics, and he figured that he was as well. He hated the idea of being an alcoholic, as this meant that he could not drink, and he still wanted to.

During the next week, Steve remained abstinent, but the following week, he had a few drinks. His wife knew nothing about it. He felt guilty about covering this up and worried that if his wife found out, it would be disastrous for their marriage. Steve wondered if he could learn how to moderate his drinking, as he greatly preferred this to abstinence. Given how much Steve used to drink, I had great reservations about whether he could learn moderation. Steve wanted to try, though, and decided that on four evenings each week, he would drink at most three drinks a couple of hours before going to bed. That would be the only time when he would drink. Before Steve implemented this plan, Sandy came to our next session because her blessing and knowledge of Steve's plan were absolutely essential. In fact, without her support, Steve's attempt to moderate his drinking wouldn't have worked. Steve's drinking was such a sore issue that, without Sandy being fully involved with Steve's plan, any drinking would have caused a huge fight between them.

In that session, although Sandy expressed her concerns, she was grateful that Steve was being honest and open with her. As Sandy learned more about his plan and the moderate drinking contract he had developed, she gave Steve her support. Steve adhered to his contract over the next three months, and sometimes he didn't even have all three drinks or drink on all four nights.

The Importance of Friends. Good friends will respect your decision, and their knowing about your plan will decrease the chance that they will offer you a drink or, without thinking, refill your glass when it is empty. Informing them about your intention may also decrease the subtle encouragement to drink more and get drunk that often happens among friends in drinking situations. This will make it easier for you to moderate your drinking. The straightforward act of informing others may also reaffirm your commitment and make it harder for you to violate your contract.

2. Moderate Drinking Rules Are Not to Be Broken

Initially, you should follow the rules you've made with no exception. Bending or changing them will lead to your drinking getting out of control again. The one exception is to change rules to ensure *less* drinking or to decrease your chances of overdrinking. As you'll see in the next chapter, you may find that you need additional structure to control your drinking successfully.

Why You Can't Change Your Rules. Until you have demonstrated good control by moderating your drinking for a period of three months, you should not change your drinking rules. Early temptations to change your rules likely indicate that you are having difficulty in holding to your contract and that your drinking is still out of control. Resist the temptation to change any rules so that you can drink in ways different from those you have already specified. Tampering with your contract is a sign that moderate drinking may not be possible for you and that abstinence may be the better way to proceed.

Paul was a 32-year-old single man who found himself drinking uncontrollably on most weekends when out with his friends from high school. He was also drinking several times during the week, so much so that he typically felt horrible the next morning, although he never missed work. He wanted to see if he could control his drinking and made a rule not to drink with his buddies, which meant that if he went out with them, he would not drink. Although he would find it difficult to see his friends and not drink, he could not fathom no longer socializing with them.

For two weeks, Paul saw his friends and didn't drink. However, in his third week of trying to control his drinking, they ended up at a bar where he had several drinks. While he knew this violated his moderate drinking contract, he felt good that he was able to limit himself to three drinks. Without informing me, he changed his contract to allow himself to drink, at most, three drinks with these friends. Two weeks later, though, he went out again with his friends, and his drinking got totally out of control.

Paul had changed his contract before he demonstrated that he could hold to its terms. Through this experience, Paul learned that he couldn't go out with his friends and drink, nor could he socialize with them when drinking was part of the picture. He changed his contract again but this time added a rule never to socialize with his high school friends in a group setting where alcohol was consumed.

When You Can Change Your Rules. You can modify your drinking rules *if you are able to hold easily to your controlled drinking contract for a period of at least three months.* A decision to modify it should be well thought out, and changes should not be made on the spur of the moment. And again, the new contract must specify clear guidelines that will govern all aspects of your drinking, just like your initial contract did. In addition, you must continue to monitor your drinking closely to see if the change in your drinking rules affects your ability to control your drinking. If it does, you must tighten the rules again and provide more structure for yourself.

Jim, a 40-year-old former client of mine, became worried when he had noticed a pattern of increased drinking over the past year, to the point that he was drinking almost every day after work and hiding it from his family. In fact, his wife, Ellen, was surprised when he told her that he thought he had a drinking problem and that he had made the decision to stop drinking. Prior to his escalated drinking, Jim had enjoyed drinking but drank only on weekends and seldom during the week. He made the decision to stop drinking and was able to achieve abstinence fairly easily.

After about three months, though, he began to miss drinking and wished he could occasionally have a glass of wine or a beer with his wife when they went out to dinner on weekends. He decided that he would attempt to moderate his drinking rather than completely abstain, and he made a drinking contract that permitted him to drink only on Friday and Saturday nights when he was out with his wife. In addition, when he drank, he would have at most two glasses of wine or two beers.

He was able to do this without difficulty, and after another three months, he wondered if he could also drink with some of his and his wife's friends. There were several couples with whom they socialized, and the couples had always drunk socially together. Until now, Jim and his wife had continued to see these other couples, but he did not drink. As he had succeeded with his current moderate drinking contract, and did not appear to struggle to hold to it, he modified his contract again. His new contract allowed him to drink still only on weekends, but he also permitted himself to drink when he socialized with their mutual friends. He also increased his consumption from two to three drinks at most. This change did not lead to any difficulties for Jim, and he continued to control his drinking successfully.

Elizabeth was a 30-year-old woman who had been married to Gary for four years and had a 2-year-old daughter. She came to see me because she was getting more and more concerned about her drinking, which she did almost every day to relax. What worried her more was her heavier drinking, which she did on the weekends with a group of her and her husband's friends. She would get quite intoxicated and started experiencing blackouts. There were even times when she embarrassed herself with her drunkenness. The next day, her friends would tell her how drunk she had been, mentioning that at times she had barely made sense when she spoke. While she knew she had been inebriated, she had no idea how truly drunk she had been. Even though her husband wasn't particularly concerned about her drinking, it bothered Elizabeth. The couple worked full-time, and Elizabeth was the primary caretaker of her daughter in the evenings when Gary attended school.

Elizabeth's parents were heavy drinkers, and she wondered whether she was an alcoholic. But over the past three weeks she had drunk on only a couple of occasions and had had two beers each time, so she wondered if she could moderate her drinking.

In our session, Elizabeth decided to drink three times per week at most, and at most she would drink three beers. She decided to limit herself to beer because she had lost control of her drinking when she drank mixed vodka drinks. She couldn't think of any situations that she needed to avoid completely so as not to lose control of her drinking, and she thought that if she stuck to beer, she could still socialize with her and her husband's friends in heavy drinking situations. She also decided to start exercising in the evenings as a way to relax.

During the next week, Elizabeth not only held to her contract, but she also didn't even have all three drinks, sometimes only two. For three months, things remained unchanged, and Elizabeth wondered if she could drink on four days if she continued to limit the number of drinks each week to nine, which was the total weekly amount in her original contract. She would still never drink more than three drinks at any one time. She revised her contract, and for seven months she held to it without problems. There were even many weeks when she didn't drink on all four days, and she continued her pattern of exercising in the evenings. She was amused at how intoxicated she used to get, and she enjoyed her new identity as a moderate drinker. Getting drunk simply became unacceptable to her.

3. The Contract Is Forever

A contract that specifies safe drinking for you is essential to maintain. Your drinking has been a problem in the past, and your vigilance is needed to ensure that you continue to moderate your drinking so that it doesn't again become excessive. Your moderate drinking contract is a reminder that you are not a social drinker. The possibility of experiencing alcohol-related problems again is real, and you must be on guard.

I have seen people moderate their drinking for years with little difficulty and increase their upper limit to four drinks without experiencing a loss of control or any alcohol-related problems. These people still, though, did not drink more than one drink per hour, and they remained mindful of the possibility of drinking too much. In addition, they typically did not drink all four drinks permitted.

I also have observed people who, after the same amount of time of successfully moderating their drinking, *occasionally* allowed themselves to drink a little more, sometimes five or six drinks, such as when they attended a get-together that lasted many hours, from the afternoon into the evening. These special events were infrequent, though. At other times these people were in control enough to continue holding to their usual limits. They also maintained other features of their moderate drinking contract, such as never drinking more than three or four times per week and remembering to pace themselves when they drank.

There are also times when, on vacation, people have allowed themselves to drink more at one time or on additional days. However, being on vacation was not a license to get drunk and let themselves return to their old ways. They remained vigilant about controlling their drinking, even though they gave themselves permission to drink somewhat more. When they returned home, they went right back to their original limits.

For these individuals, drinking in controlled ways by adhering to their contract became more or less their norm, and over time they were able to moderate their drinking with less effort. It became their way of life.

WRITING YOUR MODERATE DRINKING CONTRACT

Now you have a good sense of how to moderate your drinking. The next step is to complete your moderate drinking contract, which can be found near the end of this chapter. Since your moderate drinking contract needs to account for your own drinking pattern, here's what to do.

Get a pen, turn to the contract (or make a copy of it), and begin. Be cautious and conservative. Your drinking has been out of control, so your chance of success will improve if you are careful when setting your limits.

1. Circle the maximum number of drinks that you will ever drink in one sitting.

2. Write down the type of alcohol you will drink.

3. Circle the maximum number of times in a week you will drink.

Next, think carefully about your pattern of drinking.

4. Write down examples of the specific situations in which you have been able to control your drinking. These will be the only situations in which you can drink (your low-risk situations).

5. Write down the situations—settings, places, bars, times— in which you have lost control of your drinking. In these situations, you will never drink again (your high-risk situations).

6. Write down the social settings you need to avoid completely because, despite your best intentions, you will not be able to resist drinking too much in those settings.

7. Write down new activities and other things that you will begin to do to support your lifestyle change and help you drink less.

After you are satisfied with your moderate drinking contract, show it to the people who are most concerned about you and your drinking and try to gain their support.

KEEP A LOG OF YOUR DRINKING

Before you get started with moderation, there is one more thing I recommend that you do. On the page following the moderate drinking contract is a Log of My Drinking worksheet. You should complete this log every day until you have demonstrated that you are easily able to adhere to your moderate drinking contract and are comfortable with your ability to drink with control. The last column for "comments" is a place to note anything that could be helpful to record. For example, you may note that, on a particular day, it was challenging for you to stop at three drinks, whereas on another occasion you did so without effort.

Some people I have worked with have maintained a drinking log for years, as it kept them honest and focused on moderating their drinking. They also liked to see a visual record of their success. This log can also be useful should you have occasions where you drink too much or struggle to keep it in control. Reviewing the log might show you what went wrong and what you need to do differently to succeed.

SUMMARY

In this chapter, you learned about the seven crucial questions to answer when you develop your moderate drinking contract. You've thought long and hard about your pattern of alcohol use, and you've developed a personal moderate drinking contract that lays down rules to govern your drinking and identifies some lifestyle changes you want to make. Now is the time to put all of your energy into moderating your drinking. It's now up to you to follow your contract faithfully so that you can start to feel better about yourself and avoid any alcohol-related problems. I recommend reviewing chapter 8, which describes the general techniques of moderation that are critically important to practice. I also encourage you to keep a log of your drinking, which will train your focus on your drinking and help you ascertain what adjustments you may need to make to your contract in the event you experience any problems.

Over time, if you have been able to control your drinking without much difficulty, you may modify your moderate drinking contract, but you should do this only after you've held to it without difficulty for a period of three months. Again, the new contract needs to specify rules for your drinking just as the old one did. At all times, your drinking must fall within the limits you have specified for yourself. If it does not, you are not moderating your drinking, and you need to go back to the original moderate drinking contract that had been working for you before.

My Moderate Drinking Contract

1. When I drink, I will drink *at most*
   ☐ one drink   ☐ two drinks   ☐ three drinks   ☐ four drinks

2. I will *only* drink the following types of alcohol:
   _____

3. During a week, I will drink *at most*
   ☐ once   ☐ twice   ☐ three times   ☐ four times

4. I will *only* drink in the following situations
   (be as specific as possible): _____
   _____
   _____
   _____

5. I will *never* drink in the following situations
   (be as specific as possible): _____
   _____
   _____
   _____

6. Situations I will completely avoid
   (be as specific as possible): _____
   _____
   _____
   _____

7. Activities and interests I will engage
   in and other changes I will make: _____
   _____
   _____
   _____

Note: If I cannot successfully control my drinking, I will make the decision to stop drinking entirely.

_____
Signature and Date

Log of My Drinking

Date	Day	Type of alcohol	Setting	Time of first drink	Time of second drink	Time of third drink	Comments

CHAPTER 10

Bumps and Detours with Moderate Drinking

The road to success is always under construction.
ARNOLD PALMER

When you try to moderate your drinking, you will inevitably encounter some bumps. You may find yourself sometimes drinking more than what you agreed to in your moderate drinking contract, or you may sometimes drink more often than what you wrote in your contract. If you violate *any* rule about the amount or frequency of drinking specified in your contract, this violation is a cause for concern that needs to be addressed. While this doesn't necessarily signal that you are not able to drink moderately, it does mean that you should take a closer look at why you felt the need to drink more and consider whether abstinence should be your next step. And, regardless of how often or how much you drink, if your drinking causes you serious problems, such as finding yourself drinking and driving or getting into fights, abstinence must be considered in that case as well.

KNOWING WHETHER YOUR CONTRACT IS WORKING

In what follows I describe some problems that commonly occur when someone tries to moderate drinking and make suggestions for how to address them. If you see yourself in any of these scenarios, and if you continue to have problems even after making some adjustments to your moderate drinking contract, you should seriously consider abstinence.

Can You Succeed in Adhering to Your Contract?

The best indicator of whether moderate drinking is working for you is whether you remain in control. It's not uncommon for some problems to occur during this learning process. The trick is to learn from setbacks so that you can avoid them in the future as you continue on the path to resolving your drinking problem.

That said, you need to understand that your goal should be to succeed, especially during the first couple of months. It's not a positive sign when you have limited success during this time, and setbacks mean that abstinence is probably the better way for you to go. In my experience, having significant problems in adhering to your contract when you first try to control your drinking is a strong indicator that controlled drinking may not be possible for you.

For instance, Kevin, a 32-year-old married man, was a heavy drinker who drank almost every day. During the week, he would drink about a six-pack each night, and on the weekends, he could easily drink 10 to 15 beers in a day. He came to see me because of pressure from his wife, Debby, who was concerned about his drinking. Kevin wanted to try to moderate his drinking, so he decided that he would drink a maximum of four beers at any one sitting and would drink only three times a week. I met with Kevin and Debby, and while Debby expressed her concern about Kevin's ability to drink moderately, she was willing to support his plan. Kevin generally drank at home, but on the weekends he and Debby often went out to nightclubs, either by themselves or with friends. We discussed changing their pattern of going to clubs on the weekends, since that is where Kevin did his heaviest drinking, but Kevin believed he could control his drinking in those settings.

When I saw Kevin one week later, he reported that although he was able to drink less than he had been, he could not hold to his contract. Kevin drank four times that week and overdrank on two of those occasions, having 8 and 10 beers. As he was out at a bar when he overdrank, I suggested that Kevin either not drink at all or avoid going to bars. Kevin didn't want to hear this and stated that he simply needed to try harder.

The next week, he reported more lapses in following his contract. He had drunk on five days, not his agreed-on four. On one of those days he had only two beers, but on two days he drank seven beers at a bar. It was only then that Kevin decided that it was best not to drink at all when he went out. Unfortunately, he was unable to adhere to this decision. Over the next several weeks he decided to stop going to clubs and bars altogether, but he couldn't hold to this rule either. Only then could Kevin come to the conclusion that moderating his drinking just wasn't possible, and we worked out a plan of abstinence. If you, like Kevin, have only limited success in holding to your moderate drinking contract, particularly when you first try to do it, take it as a sign that moderate drinking is not possible for you.

How Far over Your Limit Did You Go?

If you violate your contract, ask yourself if your drinking got totally out of hand, or was it more modest? Did controlled drinking escalate to uncontrolled drinking? That is, did you find yourself downing 5 drinks when your rule was to drink no more than 3? Or did you polish off 8, 10, or 15 drinks instead of the 3? Obviously, if you are that out of control, moderate drinking is not working for you. The same can be said if you are drinking and driving or if your use of alcohol has caused you another kind of serious problem.

But if your drinking was not completely out of control, but still exceeded your self-imposed limit, it might make sense, at least for now, to continue to try moderating your drinking.

FIVE WAYS TO MAKE STICKING
TO YOUR LIMITS EASIER

1. Change Your Social Scene

Drinking is partly influenced by your social setting. When you developed your moderate drinking contract, you had to determine the types of situations that trigger you to drink excessively. These were the situations you decided not to drink in or to avoid completely.

It is also possible that you made a mistake in your contract because you overlooked what was for you a high-risk setting. If you have exceeded your drinking limit and you feel the setting might have played a role in it, consider the setting off-limits and think about whether you would do best to avoid drinking in it or to avoid it completely. Review your Log of My Drinking to see if certain situations are associated with your inability to stick to the limits you set for yourself. If you find that a situation is related, then you need to consider that situation a high-risk venue and make a change in your moderate drinking contract.

Karen, a 44-year-old successful businesswoman, first began drinking in high school. According to Karen, in high school and throughout her twenties, she only drank lightly on Friday and Saturday nights. In her thirties, perhaps influenced by the friends she socialized with, she began drinking more heavily, and on the weekends she often found herself driving home at night after having had too much to drink. In fact, one evening she was pulled over by the police, but fortunately (or unfortunately) she did not get arrested for drunk driving because she was not tested. Karen's drinking now extended to weekdays as well. This was compounded by her job, which required a fair amount of business travel and socializing with business associates. The amount of alcohol she was consuming started to concern her, and she worried about how her drinking could be affecting her health.

Karen's drinking contract specified that she would drink only on Friday and Saturday nights and *at most* once during the week, with a maximum of three drinks a night. I expressed concern about whether she could control her weekend drinking when she went out with her friends. Karen felt that she could, and she decided to talk with her friends about her plan to limit her drinking. Over the next few weeks, Karen proved me wrong and easily held to her moderate drinking contract. Feeling great about her progress, we decided that she didn't need to see me for two months, at which time we'd see how things were going.

At our next meeting, Karen reported that, to her surprise, there had been several times when she drank too much. While she had largely kept to the number of times each week she was allowed to drink, it was the amount she drank that really concerned her. On several occasions she had consumed six drinks. As we analyzed this pattern more closely, we noticed that she had been away on a business trip each time she had violated her moderate drinking contract. In the evenings, she had met her business associates in the hotel lounge, and it was during these times that she either drank too much or drank when she had planned not to.

When Karen first developed her moderate drinking contract, she didn't even consider the evenings on her business trips. She believed that she would meet her colleagues in the hotel lounge and would simply not drink or would drink on just one of the evenings. She also believed that she could limit her drinking in this situation, which proved more difficult than she initially thought. Karen revised her moderate drinking contract to specify that while on a business trip, she would go to the lounge only once during the trip. On the nights that she didn't go to the lounge, she worked out in the fitness club or stayed in her room and watched a movie or read a book. In addition, when she did go out on that one night, she would arrive later and would have, at most, one drink. This worked for Karen, and she was able to achieve success with her new moderate drinking contract.

Then there was Rob, single and 28 years old, who found that he would drink too much during his weekly poker game with friends. Instead of holding to his four-drink limit, he would commonly have five or six. Rob knew his poker game might be a problem when he developed his moderate drinking contract, yet he allowed himself this social activity. Despite his repeated attempts to control his drinking by leaving early (which he never managed to do), or by waiting to have his first drink (which he occasionally did), he was not successful and eventually made the decision to drop his poker game. He found it impossible to go there and not overdrink, so he had to modify his moderate drinking contract to make this setting off-limits.

Both Rob and Karen were able to look at their drinking patterns and, more important, to change them. The key here is to be honest with yourself and to remain focused on adhering to your contract, which must take priority over your desire to have a drink.

There are also people who, despite listing certain situations as high-risk settings to avoid, still find themselves in those social settings, where they lose control of their drinking. They eventually learn that they cannot consistently avoid those situations (and keep their drinking in control), so they choose abstinence. If you find that this occurs to you too, you'll need to give up on the idea of moderating your drinking.

2. Be Careful What You Drink

What type of alcoholic beverage were you having when your drinking turned excessive? As I explained in the last chapter, some people find that they cannot control their drinking with a certain type of alcohol. If your moderate drinking contract does not specify the type of alcohol you can drink, and you later discover by reviewing your log that one type of alcohol is problematic for you, it makes sense to modify your contract so that it specifies the beverage you are better able to control. Jason, for example, discovered that he could control his drinking by having beer only and never drinking hard liquor at all, not even in mixed drinks.

For others, the type of alcohol is irrelevant because they cannot control their alcohol use no matter what they drink. If this describes you, abstinence is your only route to recovery.

3. Limit How Much You Drink

In making your moderate drinking contract, you had to specify the maximum number of drinks you would have whenever you drank. You may have decided on four, but later you may learn that, in reality, four is too many for you. Four drinks easily turns into five or even six. Consider limiting even further how much you drink at any one time. Try to drink at most three, or even two, to see if that helps you stick to your contract. With a lower limit, moderation will be easier.

If you drink at home, limit the amount of alcohol you have on hand. For example, if you decided to drink at most three beers, keep only three beers at home and not the whole six-pack or case. Again, taking that precaution may help you moderate how much you drink. If these things don't help, the answer for you is abstinence.

4. Slow Down Your Drinking

As I mentioned in the last chapter, I recommend that you try to make one drink last for one hour or at least for 45 minutes. Drinking too quickly can cause you to have too many drinks.

Review your drinking log to see how quickly you had your second or third drink after having your first. If you find that you had your second drink shortly after your first, or a third drink a short time after your second, remember to slow down your drinking by making each drink last close to one hour. If you can't do it, that's a sign that abstinence may be the better way to proceed. You should also remember that you can take a break after finishing a drink before you have another. This will also help you slow down your drinking and reduce the number of drinks that you have.

5. Shorten the Window of Your Drinking

Regardless of the setting you drink in, the longer you have to drink, the greater your chance of drinking too much becomes. For example, if you are at a get-together that begins at three o'clock and doesn't end until nine at night, your chance of overdrinking is greater than if the get-together lasted only four hours. Similarly, even when you are at home, if your drinking begins at five o'clock and you go to bed at nine, the possibility of your overdrinking is greater than if you began to drink at seven o'clock.

When reviewing her drinking log, Jane found that if she opened a bottle of wine right when she got home from work at half past five o'clock, she often drank most, if not all, of the bottle. However, if she waited until seven o'clock or later, she was able to slow herself down and have only two glasses. Eric discovered that when he and his wife got together with other couples, he could better control his drinking if he waited to have his first drink after one or two hours had passed instead of immediately having a drink.

If you find yourself drinking more than what you specified in your contract, review the times you began to drink and the length of time you allowed yourself to drink. If you notice that you are giving yourself large windows of time in which to drink, start drinking later in the day to see whether shrinking your window for drinking helps you control your consumption. If it does not, you may need to consider abstinence.

DO YOU DRINK MORE OFTEN THAN THE RULE IN YOUR CONTRACT?

Even if your drinking does not get totally out of control on any one occasion, you may still be violating your contract by drinking more often than you specified you would. For instance, instead of drinking three times per week, you may drink four, five, or six times.

Think about your inability to comply with your moderate drinking contract. Do you often drink more frequently than your rule specifies, or is this an occasional occurrence? An occasional violation means that your drinking exceeds the rule a few times a year. A frequent violation is anything more, whether it be monthly or weekly. Simply put, you cannot permit yourself to exceed the limits you set. A slipup once, twice, or even three times a year is acceptable—you are human after all—provided that your drinking did not cause you serious difficulties. Any more than that and you should consider abstinence.

TWO WAYS TO AVOID DRINKING TOO OFTEN

1. Think about and Change Your Surroundings

Just as the physical and social setting in which you drink is important in limiting the amount of alcohol you drink at a time, the same principle applies to the number of times you drink each week. Even if your drinking does not exceed your limit in terms of the amount, if you do find yourself drinking more often than you specified, you should identify when you increased your frequency.

Brad, 26 years old and single, had decided that he was only going to drink three times each week, but he found that he regularly drank five or six times weekly. When he looked closely at this pattern, he discovered that he tended to drink whenever he got together with a certain group of friends after work. He was also in a bowling league where the members always drank, and this made it easy for him to exceed his limit of drinking three times per week. He eventually made the decision to quit his bowling league and see his drinking buddies less often. While Brad's friends were important to him, as was his bowling, his drinking problem was an even higher priority.

Brenda, a single mom, found that her drinking increased from three times a week to four or five times if alcohol was available at her house. Her leisure time involved simply winding down at home after work, and while she couldn't change that, she could change having a lot of alcohol readily available to her in this situation. She decided to keep a limited amount of alcohol at home only on the days when she allowed herself to drink, and this limit on supply helped her stick to her three-day-per-week rule.

Mike, a 34-year-old single man, wanted to limit his drinking to three times per week but instead found himself drinking four or five times. His pattern was to come home from work and unwind in his den with the television on, which was his element. He decided to join a fitness center where he would go straight from work and then, after his workout, go home. That change to his routine enabled him to hold to his three-day limit.

If your own drinking exceeds your rule for how often you can drink, try to figure out why this is happening. There are, no doubt, situations you need to alter or avoid that you hadn't thought about when you made your contract, and now is the time to make these changes. If you still continue to drink too often no matter how you try to modify your contract, abstinence will be your best and only choice. It is just that simple.

2. Limit How Often You Drink

You may also need to reevaluate the number of times each week you allow yourself to drink. The maximum number of days anyone should drink in a week is four, and drinking on four days may not provide you enough time without drinking. Four days easily can grow to five or six. If you decided to drink on four days but are having trouble holding to this limit, try decreasing your maximum to two or three. Further restriction may help you moderate your drinking.

Mark, for instance, originally decided that he would drink on Friday and Saturday nights and twice during the week. However, before long, he found himself drinking Thursday through Sunday and then occasionally on other weekdays as well. For him, reducing the number of times he could drink to two gave him the bounds he needed.

TAKE THE SUGGESTED BREAK FROM DRINKING

In chapter 8, where I reviewed some general techniques to moderate drinking, I suggested taking a one-month or two-week break from drinking before starting to drink moderately. Or if that seems too long, take at least one week off. That interruption will help break your pattern of drinking. Swearing off alcohol for a while can give you confidence that you do not need to drink and an opportunity to do other things with your time that do not include drinking. It also can strengthen your commitment to change, as deciding to abstain even temporarily forces you to admit with more conviction the need to address your drinking.

If you did not take a break from drinking and find yourself struggling to control it, I strongly encourage you to start over. Take the recommended break from drinking, see what it is like not to drink at all, and then restart your rule-bound moderation. The temporary break may give you much insight into what you need to do to better control your drinking. You may discover when and where you crave alcohol the most, so those will be the times and situations you need to regulate. With this insight, you should rewrite your moderate drinking contract to see whether that modification enables you to succeed. If that does not help, abstinence will be your better choice.

LIMITING ALCOHOL ISN'T ALWAYS EASY

If you have successfully moderated your intake, how difficult is it to do? Do you still enjoy drinking, or does the hassle of limiting your intake make drinking no longer pleasurable? Is it a struggle to avoid daily drinking or to reduce your drinking to only three or four times a week? Do you find yourself wanting to drink more than you are allowed? Are you wondering if it is worth the effort and struggle?

For some people, moderating drinking is not a constant effort, and for some, it may even be fairly easy to do. However, if this is not the case for you, and moderating alcohol intake becomes an unpleasant experience, it makes sense for you to try abstinence. Why? Because moderating your drinking should not be unpleasant. The benefits to your life that result from drinking less should start to outweigh and outnumber the pleasures of immoderate drinking that previously came coupled with problems. Think long and hard about this. Remember, your only choices are moderation or abstinence. Drinking more is not an option.

MODERATION DOESN'T ALWAYS WORK, AND THAT'S OKAY

A common scenario among problem drinkers is the difficulty they have acknowledging that they cannot moderate their drinking. You may try and try to limit your alcohol consumption but with only limited success. You may wish to be like those who can drink without problems, but that is all it is: *a wish.*

When you finally believe that controlling your drinking is not possible and is only a wish, that is when you're on the road to getting better. Moderate drinking may not have succeeded in the way you first thought and hoped it would. But it has succeeded nonetheless because it proved to you that your use of alcohol cannot be moderated and that abstinence needs to be the way you resolve your alcohol problem. You have learned something very important about yourself.

IT COMES DOWN TO MODERATION OR ABSTINENCE

The decision to give up on moderate drinking and pursue instead a course of abstinence is a tough one. *But this is what you need to do if you want alcohol to stop interfering with your life.* The evidence is clear: if alcohol continues to hurt you, even though you are trying your best to moderate your drinking, you need to give it up entirely.

Some people just cannot moderate their drinking, despite their best efforts. Don't get down on yourself. Accept this fact, and I promise you that it won't be long before you see how true this advice is.

Make the decision to stop drinking completely and see how your life improves.

Sean was a 32-year-old married man and father of 1-year-old twins. Sean had been a "heavy partyer" in high school and in his twenties. He could easily drink 15 beers in the course of an evening and sometimes even more. He and his friends were all into heavy drinking, and on many nights they congregated at one of several local bars, drinking quite heavily and staying out late. Prior to getting married, Sean wasn't particularly concerned about his drinking, as he had few other responsibilities and partying was an important part of his life.

Now, five years into his marriage, Sean had slowed down his drinking, but he still drank heavily at the bars on many nights, sometimes with his wife, Ann, who was a light drinker, and at other times without her. After Ann gave birth to their twins, Sean's heavy drinking began to become more of an issue. While Ann stayed home caring for their children, Sean was out drinking. There were times on the weekends when Sean got so drunk that he was incapable of assisting Ann with childcare the next day. When his drinking started to affect his relationship with Ann, Sean got concerned.

He drew the line at abstinence and preferred to try to moderate his drinking. He decided that he would drink at most four beers per occasion and would drink only on Friday and Saturday nights and once during the week. He still wanted to be able to drink with his friends at the local bars, and he thought he could control his drinking there.

The next week, Sean reported that his success had been mixed. While he drank only three times, one of those times he drank way too much at the bar and got home very late, which caused an argument with Ann. However, on a weekend night out at the bar with Ann, he was able to limit his drinking. So he revised his contract to allow himself to drink at bars only when Ann was with him. He would still go to bars by himself, but those times he would not drink alcohol.

This revision, unfortunately, didn't work for long. Sean started drinking in bars without Ann and ended up getting drunk and getting home late. He then decided that he would never go to a bar without Ann, and he revised his contract to reflect this. That, too, did not work because after going out with Ann and drinking a little too much, he would return home with her and then immediately head out again and get inebriated.

Even after all this, Sean still would not consider abstinence. As a last-ditch effort at moderation, he decided that the *only* time he would ever drink was when he went out to dinner with Ann. At restaurants they often would split a bottle of wine, and that never seemed to present a problem for him. He also decided that he would never go to another bar, as he simply could not control his drinking in that setting. We discussed the idea of his doing some limited drinking while at home, but Sean never drank at home and had no desire to start. So his contract was now modified so that he was only permitted to drink on the weekends when out to dinner with Ann (where they would split one bottle of wine) and never would he go to a bar alone or with friends.

Despite this newly drafted contract, over the next couple of months, Sean reverted to going to bars occasionally and getting extremely intoxicated. I'm happy to say, though, that Sean finally admitted to himself that the only way he was ever going to solve his drinking problem was abstinence. After he made this decision, his life began to improve.

HOW BUMPS AND DETOURS CAN WORK
TO YOUR ADVANTAGE

The process of trying to moderate your drinking may be something you needed to do. Discovering that you can't drink moderately is actually a positive development. You learned a lot about yourself and your relationship to alcohol, and you now know that you need to stop drinking completely to resolve your drinking problem. If you didn't go through this process, you would always wonder if you could moderate your drinking, and this would make it difficult for you to commit to abstinence. So your journey has given you self-knowledge and has solidified in your mind what you now must do—achieve abstinence from alcohol.

While moderating drinking represents a lifestyle change, quitting drinking is an even bigger one. But try not to feel overwhelmed. Many, many people learn to quit drinking and still love life. In fact, many have learned to love life even more without drinking—and so will you. I have even heard some say that learning to live life without alcohol was the best thing that ever happened to them. So don't be scared by what you are facing. Instead, view it as a new journey and an opportunity for growth.

SUMMARY

You know now whether or not moderation is working for you. If you encountered some bumps along the way but have learned from these experiences and modified your drinking contract to enable you to succeed, that's great! In fact, some bumps are inevitable and give you insight into your pattern of drinking and what traps you need to be on guard for. The key is learning from these experiences so that you don't step into the same traps over and over.

However, if you keep experiencing bumps and your drinking problem continues no matter how you modify your contract, you have learned that abstinence needs to be your next step. And that's okay. The next four chapters will help you stop drinking entirely.

Facts do not cease to exist because they are ignored.
ALDOUS HUXLEY

PART IV

Quitting Drinking and Staying Sober

CHAPTER 11

Managing Your Thoughts to Quit Drinking

Self-discipline begins with the mastery of your thoughts. If you don't control what you think, you can't control what you do. Simply, self-discipline enables you to think first and act afterward.

NAPOLEON HILL

I'm sure that your decision to stop drinking has not been easy. Drinking has been an important part of your life, and the idea of quitting may be a little scary. But now you realize that you cannot moderate your drinking and that abstinence is the only way to stop alcohol from ruining your life. You may even have tried to moderate your drinking by reading this book and were not successful. Regardless of how you reached the decision to abstain from alcohol, you must now learn to avoid drinking and commit yourself to making this a reality.

There are many proven techniques that will help you not take that first drink and that will make quitting alcohol much less stressful. You can learn these techniques in the privacy of your home rather than by going to AA or other self-help meetings, psychiatrists, psychologists, alcohol counselors, or more intensive treatment programs. Whether you consider your drinking problem a disease or a bad habit does not matter, as these techniques will help you regardless of how you understand why you can't control your drinking. The only things that matter are your commitment and desire to stop drinking.

The fact that you know you need to abstain from alcohol permanently to resolve your drinking problem suggests that your problem with alcohol is somewhat serious. As I mentioned in chapter 6, alcohol can damage your body, and I would strongly encourage you to see your doctor to get checked out. In the event that you have any medical conditions caused or worsened by your drinking, you should know so that you can get them treated. In addition, some people with a more severe alcohol problem have emotional problems as well, whether these are feelings of anxiety, extreme moodiness, or just feeling down in the dumps. These emotional problems may have preceded their drinking problem or been caused by it. Regardless, if these problems are not treated, they can make the process of getting sober more difficult. So, if you experience these kinds of feelings, talk with your doctor about them. Your doctor can refer you for psychological counseling, which I review in chapter 17, or to a psychiatrist who can evaluate your need for psychiatric medication, which I review in chapter 18. While you may not need medication, it is a good idea for you to get checked out so that you know for certain. Remember, too, that using alcohol to cope will not help you in the long run and will prevent you from getting better. With that being said, let's now consider ways for you to think about your alcohol problem that will make the process of quitting alcohol easier.

YOU ARE NOT ALONE

The idea of no longer drinking is probably unsettling to you. Quitting alcohol will be a major change in the way you live your life, and you may even believe that you are in an extreme minority. The idea that most everyone drinks, except you and others who have made the decision to stop, can make you feel isolated and different. But you shouldn't think that you are missing out on something by abstaining. If drinking was so great, why did it cause you so much grief? You're quitting so that you *won't* miss out on anything in life.

If you're falling into the familiar trap of thinking that most everyone drinks but you, that's because alcohol has been central to most of your social activities for much of your life. You may be surprised to learn that many, many people do not drink at all. When people in the United States are asked about their alcohol use, about 29 percent of adults 18 years of age and older report that they have not drunk alcohol in the past year, and 43 percent report not drinking in the past month. As you enter a sober lifestyle, you'll experience this first-hand. These nondrinkers live fulfilled and happy lives. Not drinking is simply a lifestyle choice; it does not need to be as big of an issue as you may think. Sure, you need to adjust to this, as it represents a big change for you, but it is a choice you won't regret making. So let's get on with it. Stopping drinking is not easy, but drinking the way you have hasn't been easy either. Remember that you aren't alone. Like others, you will learn to enjoy life without drinking.

NOT TO DRINK: YOUR NUMBER ONE PRIORITY

Make Not Drinking Your Daily Thought

Every day, take the time to remember that you are trying to change your life by not taking even one drink. When you wake up every morning, remind yourself of this by saying out loud, "*Today* I am choosing not to drink." This is your first step to sobriety. It is not as though you *can't* drink. Rather, it is your choice not to drink. Many people I have worked with have found remembering that it is a choice to be very helpful. No one wants to be told what they can or cannot do, and that is probably true for you. No one is telling you that you cannot drink. You are choosing not to drink to feel healthier and to feel better about your life.

You'll succeed if you remember to keep your decision not to drink in the forefront of your mind. You must live and breathe this thought, all day and every day. Abstinence is your goal for today. Then, plan your day with activities that do not include drinking. Here's how.

Planning a Life without Alcohol

When you first stop drinking, plan your day around avoiding all alcohol-related activities. Be prepared, anticipate, carefully evaluate, and avoid any situation that can potentially endanger your abstinence.

For example, if your friends suggest stopping off for a drink after work, don't try to convince yourself that you can go with them and not drink. Instead, find a pleasant way to decline the invitation. If you are invited to play cards or to attend a barbecue, and you believe that drinking will be a part of the social setting, you should also decline because of the possibility that you might be tempted to drink. Making the decision to avoid former problem situations is not easy, and you will not be able to foresee every temptation. If your goal of not drinking is your number one thought, however, you will be prepared to make these decisions.

As you become more comfortable in your new role as a non-drinker, you'll be able to participate in more activities where alcohol is served. But for now, it's best to avoid these activities altogether.

Be Prepared with Excuses

You may want to think in advance about what to say when you decline an invitation. At times you may feel comfortable saying that you are trying to stop drinking and that you're turning down the offer because you would be too tempted to drink. In other situations you may feel more comfortable offering the excuse of having other plans or other things to do. Feel free to say different things to different people depending on how well you know them or the type of relationship you have with them. There is no right or wrong way to decline; just say what feels right for you at the time. Your explanation may change as you grow more comfortable with your decision not to drink.

As you grow accustomed to being a nondrinker in places where alcohol is available, you should also be prepared with what to say when you turn down a drink. At times, people may feel comfortable stating that they do not drink, whereas in other situations those same people might say that their stomach is upset, they are taking a medication that does not mix with alcohol, they simply do not feel like drinking, they have to drive, or they are feeling tired. Again, there is no right or wrong response, and you should say what feels right given the circumstance and your comfort level.

Focus on the Benefits of Not Drinking

It is important to try not to dwell on what you are not doing or what you think you are missing. Instead, focus on the positive benefits of no longer drinking and how your life is improving (you're not fighting with your spouse; you're alert and prepared at the office; you're saving money by not buying alcohol; you feel better physically; you have less guilt; you're no longer drinking and driving).

In chapter 4, you thought about and wrote down all of the pros to changing your relationship to alcohol. Now is the time to recall what these are. Remembering the benefits of sobriety will keep you concentrated on why you have made the decision to stop drinking.

ONE DAY AT A TIME

Alcoholics Anonymous encourages taking things "one day at a time," and this is a good strategy for you, too. Here's how it works: think about not drinking for *today* and for *today only*. This strategy is much more manageable than thinking about not drinking for the rest of your life, which may be overwhelming for you right now. Instead, try to live with the thought "I am not drinking today," and then do everything in your power not to drink between morning and bedtime. You can even break it down into smaller chunks of time if you need to. For example, if your pattern was to go for a drink after work, you can tell yourself, "tonight, for the next five hours, I am not going to drink."

One-day-at-a-time thinking also can be useful when you encounter other difficult situations in your life, including financial hardship, a relationship breakup, a medical problem, or other troubles. Particularly when you first abstain from alcohol, problems may feel overwhelming and impossible to bear without a drink. This is because you probably have not developed all of the coping skills you need to since you used to use alcohol as a way to cope. During these times it can be helpful to remember that all you really need to do is get through the day.

Less Is More: Small Steps Lead to Big Changes
Again, you can break your periods of abstinence into even smaller units, such as one hour at a time or even minutes at a time. If you segment your time this way, it will be much easier for you to deal with almost any temptation to take a drink. Here's why: The shorter the time, the easier it is to avoid temptation for almost any compulsive activity, whether it is smoking, eating unhealthy food, or drinking alcohol. Keeping this up for the rest of your life may seem impossible, but the next hour or the next half hour is easily doable and sometimes long enough for the urge to drink to pass. And that's the whole point: clear one small hurdle at a time.

I have often used the analogy of imagining that you have not eaten for 24 hours and are very hungry. Suddenly, a nice plate of food is placed before you, and you are told that you cannot touch it for four hours. That would be really hard to do. However, if I asked you to wait 15 minutes to eat, I am sure you'd find that much easier to do. If you need to, breaking down not drinking into manageable units of time is the way to go.

For instance, Bob found that "keeping it in the day" was the main thing he needed to do to remain abstinent. "All I need to remember is to not drink today . . . and only today. Tomorrow isn't anything I need to worry or think about. Tomorrow turns into today, and I only think about that when it comes and never before."

You may question this one-day-at-a-time philosophy and think that it is childlike and that long-range planning is important. It is true that many goals are only achieved by taking into account the far horizon (saving money for retirement, buying a home, and setting up a business are some examples). However, when it comes to stopping a compulsive activity like drinking, the one-day-at-a-time philosophy really works.

For example, let's assume that it is August, and you have decided to stop drinking. Don't think now about not being able to drink when you celebrate Thanksgiving or New Year's Eve or attend your friend's bachelor party next year. That kind of thinking will overwhelm you and bring you down. Instead, deal with today and cope with these future events as they happen. You will probably find that when those events come around, not drinking will be no big deal.

Stay in the Present

Remember that you will think and feel differently in the future than you do now. While the idea of not being able to drink on New Year's Eve might sound dreadful in August, when New Year's Eve comes, and you have some abstinence under your belt and have learned to enjoy your life without needing a drink, not drinking may not even be an issue. Worry about and think about tomorrow only when tomorrow comes . . . and never before.

Scott stopped drinking in September and was worried about celebrating Christmas with his family. Getting together for Christmas was the family tradition, and everyone drank heavily at that time. In October, Scott just didn't know how he was going to handle this. Should he even go? If he didn't go, how would his family feel? Could he go and not drink? He even wondered if he could enjoy Christmas at all without drinking. Scott finally decided that he would worry about this in two months, and in the meantime he simply focused on not drinking in the present. And when Christmas arrived, he discovered that celebrating it was no longer a big issue. He decided to stop by his family's home for a short period of time, and he spent most of the evening with his wife, Sarah, starting a new tradition—driving around to see the Christmas lights and then having a quiet, romantic evening at home.

Feeling Better Happens One Day at a Time

Remember that once you stop drinking, it will take time before you begin to feel better. So don't be discouraged if your life doesn't turn around immediately after you stop drinking.

Even though your drinking has ended, the damage that alcohol has done to you may be present for a long time. Your relationships may still be filled with tension and conflict. You may continue to experience difficulties at work, or you may be dealing with drink-related legal problems. Or perhaps you are seeing your life with a clear head for the first time in a long time, and you do not like what you see. Now is the time you must be strong, because any of these difficulties or disappointments can lead you back to drinking. But don't retreat. Drinking may seem like the easier option, but it's not. Over time, if you drink, your problems will only compound, your health will suffer, and your relationships will deteriorate. Staying abstinent is the best choice. The harder choice to make now, maybe, but well worth it for a happy, healthy future.

You may also experience what is called a protracted withdrawal syndrome, in which you continue to feel a little off and not like yourself even after any acute withdrawal from alcohol has passed. During this time, your sleep can be disturbed, and you can feel tired, have low energy, and can even sometimes feel a little anxious or depressed. Not everyone experiences these feelings, but for some, this can be another reason why you do not immediately feel better. Again, though, don't be discouraged. Remember that you will begin to feel better in time and these feelings will pass if you keep focused on maintaining abstinence.

Recovering from a drinking problem occurs one day at a time. It will take time to get your life to where you would like it to be. If you have been drinking for 20 years, it may take more than a few weeks, or even a few months, to begin to feel really good about your life, but things will get a bit better every day.

Try not to get frustrated. You have made the commitment not to drink. Success will be within your grasp if you keep that priority clear in your mind and remember that you *will* begin to feel better, but only one day at a time.

Time Is a Healer

It may sound like a cliché, but time is an amazing healer. What seems unbearable now will not be so in the future. In time, you will develop additional coping skills and a greater ability to deal with whatever happens. Meeting difficulties one day at a time and just getting through the day can often be enormously useful. Deal with your future when it comes and not before.

NEVER FORGET THE CONSEQUENCES OF YOUR DRINKING

Although some parts of drinking were enjoyable, other parts had a destructive impact on your life. *Wanting to avoid the consequences of drinking is one of the primary reasons you decided to do something about your drinking problem.* Always remain mindful of the pain your drinking has caused and will continue to cause you if you return to it.

It is common for ex-drinkers to minimize the extent of their past drinking. They begin to think that their problem wasn't so bad. When they crave a drink, they may actually forget about their past difficulties. The mind has an amazing ability to forget pain and to play tricks on us. Don't let this happen to you.

Write a List of Harmful Consequences and Review It Daily

Write a list of the harm drinking has caused you and others. Spend time thinking of all of the ways drinking has hurt you, affected your sense of self and self-esteem, or hurt your relationships with others. Keep this list handy for quick reference, and review it daily to keep the pain fresh in your mind. You should also often reread the cons of your drinking from the Pros and Cons of My Drinking exercise that you completed in chapter 4. Doing this will keep you focused on the reasons why you have decided to stop drinking.

This exercise is not meant to make you feel bad; rather, it is meant to help you remember why you made the commitment to drink no more. The harm and bad feelings caused by your past drinking must remain alive in your mind. If you begin to forget why you stopped drinking, this list can be a useful reminder to you. Particularly when you first stop drinking, make it a *daily habit* to review this list to stay focused on why you are no longer drinking and recall what will occur if you start drinking again.

Write a Goodbye Letter to Alcohol

It can also be helpful to write a "goodbye letter" to alcohol. You have had a close relationship to alcohol; it has been an important part of your life. There are parts of drinking that you have enjoyed. At the same time, alcohol has caused you way too many problems. You need to mourn the loss of alcohol from your life, just like you may have needed to mourn the loss of other important things in your life.

In this letter, tell alcohol all of the reasons why you have decided to end your relationship with it. Think of the numerous ways that alcohol has negatively affected your life, and let alcohol know that you no longer wish to maintain this relationship. Although parts of drinking have been pleasurable, the negative aspects of drinking dwarf any of the positive ones. Now is the time you must say goodbye to alcohol. Once you've written the letter, you should review it often to keep your reasons for not drinking fresh in your mind. You should reread it especially if you ever begin to think about drinking again.

Always Keep in Mind the Benefits of Not Drinking

While the pain your drinking has caused you and others in your life is a key factor in your decision not to drink, the benefits you will achieve by not drinking must also be remembered. You must keep in mind the vision you want for yourself and how no longer drinking will enable you to reach your goals. *Wanting to have a better life is the other primary reason why you have made the decision to change your relationship to alcohol.*

Write a List of Benefits of Not Drinking and Review It Daily
Write a list of all the ways your commitment to abstinence will enhance your life. Think about your life goals, your health, what you want to achieve, how your relationships with others will improve, and how not drinking will improve your self-esteem and self-concept. Review this daily, as it will help keep you focused on your decision to stop drinking. Reread what you wrote for the Pros and Cons of My Drinking and Pros and Cons of My Changing exercises and focus on the cons of drinking and pros of changing. How your life will improve by abstaining from alcohol must always be kept in your mind.

ABSTINENCE IS ABSTINENCE—FOREVER

You already know that you can't moderate your drinking and that abstinence is the only way to recover from your drinking problem. You've probably tried dozens of times, if not more, to control your drinking, and because you couldn't do this, you're now committed to staying sober. So why am I telling you that abstinence is abstinence—forever? You know this, right? Here's why: After a period of successful abstinence, it is *extremely* common for people to begin to think they can drink again because they believe that it will be different this time around.

You can admit that you drank too much in the past and lost control of your drinking, but this time, after a period of abstinence as your proof, you may start to believe that you will be able to control your drinking and won't allow it to take over your life again. You tell yourself that, with all you have learned in your sobriety, you will be able to drink safely and will *never* allow yourself to drink too much. This time, you will be careful and control your drinking. Wrong!

What Is One Drink to an Ex-drinker?
Maybe you tell yourself that you will have *just one drink.* While you know that this holds the potential for difficulties, you believe that

having just one drink won't hurt and will not escalate into more drinking. At the moment, you want to have a drink, and at the moment, you believe that it will cause no harm. After all, what's one drink?

Even One Drink Is Too Much

You've already proved to yourself that you cannot moderate your alcohol consumption, so one drink is never an option for you. In fact, for you, *any drinking has the potential and will likely, if not definitely, lead to too much drinking.* Losing your commitment not to drink, and "forgetting" that you cannot drink any alcohol safely, can lead you back to excessive drinking. Beware. Once the door to your old behavior is ajar, it can quickly open all the way, and your drinking will again become excessive. Whatever your good intentions, you need to remember that this time will not be different. You are not able to moderate your drinking, and one drink is too much.

You May Want to Drink

Do not be surprised if there are days when you will want to drink. *This is normal and you should expect this.* As I have written, your decision to stop drinking has nothing to do with your dislike of alcohol. You like to drink, and if you could control your use of alcohol so that it caused you no difficulty, you would continue to drink and would not be reading this chapter.

Accept the Thought and Think It Through

If such a thought arises, and it likely will, simply accept that this is to be expected, and tell yourself, "Of course I want to drink, but I can choose not to drink." Realize that such a thought is normal and do not fall into its trap. Again, remember the negative impact that drinking will have on your life and the positive effect that maintaining abstinence will have for you. Instead of thinking about how much you would like to drink, try to distract your mind, and you will find that it passes.

THERE'S NEVER A GOOD REASON TO DRINK

One of the easiest things to find is a reason to drink. Drinking can be justified for almost any reason:

- It was a good day.

- It was a bad day.

- It was a sunny day.

- It was a rainy day.

- You had a stressful day at work.

- You successfully closed on a deal you had been working on for months.

- Your favorite team won the Super Bowl.

- Your favorite team lost the Super Bowl.

It doesn't matter. If you want to drink, you can always find a reason. However, a *reason* to drink is simply an *excuse* to drink. In reality, there is never a reason to drink, and you need to be mindful that your brain will play tricks on you and try to convince you that there is.

Even Terrible Events Aren't Reasons to Drink

Life is filled with its ups and downs. On certain days, everything works out well, yet on other days, Murphy's law prevails. Nothing goes right, and you may feel angry, frustrated, or resentful. When bad things happen and you feel angry, down, resentful, frustrated, or anxious, it's very tempting to tell yourself that you *deserve* a drink.

This is not in any way meant to minimize bad experiences such as a relationship breakup, getting diagnosed with a serious illness, or the death of someone close to you. Neither do I want to take lightly the feelings of intense anxiety or depression that some people experience when trying to stay sober and that may be related to events in their lives. However, no matter what happens or what you experience, *there is never a good reason for you to drink.* While you may believe that drinking can help you in the short term, it will only hurt you in the long term and eventually will make everything worse. Take Bob, who internalized a "zero-tolerance" policy. Regardless of what happened in his life, there was no place for drinking because he knew that "drinking would just mess everything up." Certainly, if you continue to be bothered by painful feelings, there are outside resources to help you, which I review in part V of this book. Drinking, however, is not one of them.

SUMMARY

You now know a lot of ways to think about your decision of abstinence that will make it easier for you not to drink. In large part, your thoughts control your behavior, so you need to remember that and incorporate these strategies into your daily thinking. It isn't easy to change our usual and automatic ways of thinking, so it is important that you practice the following:

- Remember that many people do not drink. You are not alone.
- Make no longer drinking your number one priority.
- Stop drinking one day at a time, or even an hour at a time, and worry about the future only when it comes.
- Focus on and never forget the consequences of your drinking.
- Focus on and never forget the benefits of not drinking and how that will improve your life.
- Keep in mind that one drink is too much, as it will open the door to out-of-control drinking. Abstinence is abstinence—forever.
- Wanting to drink is normal. Do not be seduced by this thought.
- A reason to drink is only an excuse to drink. There is never a good reason to drink.

CHAPTER 12

What You Must Do
to Quit Drinking

Activity is contagious.
RALPH WALDO EMERSON

To stop drinking, you will have to change not just the way you think but also some of your behaviors. By this, I mean that you need to fill the gap in your life left by alcohol. You probably never realized how much of your day was either spent drinking or wasted because you were unable to function. The extra time you now have will be quite an adjustment, and you need to learn to fill it with things other than drinking, such as catching up with old friends, hanging out with your partner, playing with your kids, or finding a new hobby.

BOREDOM CAN LEAD BACK TO DRINKING

When you first stop drinking, it's common to feel like a fish out of water. You probably won't know what to do with yourself. This happens either because your drinking had replaced other previously familiar, pleasurable activities or because you never even developed other leisure activities since drinking was the central focus of your life. Most of your social and leisure activities may have involved drinking, so now you find that you can no longer participate in some activities that were a part of your drinking life (including, perhaps, spending time in bars, dart games, card games, playing golf, bowling, watching a football game, and hanging out with particular friends), and this can make you feel bored. The danger is that your life can begin to seem dull and empty, which may lead you back to drinking. In fact, boredom is a big reason why people return to drinking after a period of abstinence. To stay the course and not drink, you must fill the void.

THE DRY DRUNK

If you are able to stop drinking, yet don't fill the gap left by alcohol, you will feel miserable, bored, and empty and so won't be happy about not drinking. And that's not good. The term *dry drunk* refers to an individual who is no longer drinking but who has not made any lifestyle changes. The dry drunk feels resentful about not drinking and negative about life and, over time, may return to drinking. Dry drunks exhibit the same unattractive behaviors as do active drinkers, except now the behaviors aren't triggered by having a drink. Dry drunks are not fun to be around. You need to make serious lifestyle changes so that you will love being alive again and have an optimistic outlook on life. You must regain your ability to laugh, love, plan for the future, and make time for friends and family. True recovery is the enjoyment of life without alcohol.

Think of your life as a pie. Alcohol, a big slice of that pie, has been cut out and removed. If you have the feeling that a big piece of your life is missing, you will feel partly empty and bored. If you don't fill the void, you may remain abstinent, but you won't enjoy it. The key is discovering that your life is even more fulfilling and fun without drinking. It is critical that you keep busy, structure your days, and find fun things to do that don't include drinking in order to avoid becoming a dry drunk or returning to drinking.

STRUCTURE YOUR DAY AND MAKE PLANS

Every day, make a plan for the next day. Fill the times of the day when you used to drink with alcohol-free events. There are probably things you always wanted to do, places to see, or projects around the house that were not possible when drinking consumed your leisure time. Even something as simple as reading a book or going to a movie can stimulate you and take your mind off alcohol. Plan ahead and hold to that plan. Faithfully staying to your schedule (as long as it doesn't include activities you associate with drinking) decreases your chances of returning to alcohol.

Filling in the Times When You Used to Drink

For example, let's assume you work from nine to five o'clock, and before abstinence you commonly drank after work. The question is, What will you do from the time work ends until bedtime? That's where planning ahead comes in. You should know what you are going to do that evening. Make it a point never to be in the situation of leaving work with no plans for the evening. These plans can be as simple as a going to the supermarket, browsing a bookstore, taking a walk or jog, hitting the health club, watching a particular TV program, or cooking yourself (or your family) a nice meal. Having plans doesn't mean you need to attend a concert or play or sports event every night. The goal is to do something that gives you pleasure so that you enjoy your life more than the drinking life you are leaving behind.

As I review in detail in chapter 15, one reason many people find support groups such as Alcoholics Anonymous helpful is that attending meetings helps to fill those evenings when they have nothing to do. There, you can learn some useful tips for how to remain abstinent while you meet other people, and it gives you a social activity that doesn't involve drinking.

Weekends

For many people, weekends can be the toughest times. If you work during the week, the weekends can seem very long. It is also likely that your weekends were often filled with drinking. Especially when you first stop drinking, ensure that you have plans for weekends. Plan to take a scenic drive or visit someplace familiar or new that will take up much of the day. Maybe fill a chunk of the day running errands and then go the movies or listen to a lecture. Anything that interests you will help to fill the day and keep your mind off drinking.

DEVELOP NEW LEISURE ACTIVITIES

This is also a great time to begin some activities that you always wanted to do but didn't because drinking got in the way. Maybe you always wanted to learn how to scuba dive, take art lessons, or take a French course. Or maybe learning how to ski or play tennis or a musical instrument sounds fun to you. There is a whole world out there to enjoy, and there is no better time to start than now.

Why fill your time with drinking when you can have more fun doing other things? Here are more suggestions to help jump-start your thinking:

- visit a museum

- take a walk along the beach

- go to the library

- read a book

- take up a martial art

- learn to dance

- make gourmet dinners

- see a movie

- take up kickboxing

- build a piece of furniture
- enroll in a pottery class
- go parachuting
- learn to knit
- take a walk in the woods
- try your hand at doing some artwork
- join a garden club
- take up stargazing
- join a community theater group
- take singing lessons
- go whitewater rafting, canoeing, or kayaking
- take up photography

A great resource for thinking about and getting involved in new leisure activities is the online app Meetup. By searching meetups near you, you will discover many different interest groups gathering where you can do things with people who have the same interests as you. If you engage in activities and meet new people, you will have less time to think about drinking and find other life interests (and friends) that are fun and stimulating and don't take place in a bar or require alcohol to take part.

PHYSICAL ACTIVITY

Physical activity is great for many reasons. It not only gets you in shape, but it also provides you with a sense of accomplishment, gives you confidence, and improves your self-esteem. It is also something you can do at any time of the day, any day, to keep busy. There are many different types of physical activity to choose from, many of which you can do yourself at home. Yoga, calisthenics, running, walking, tennis, horseback riding, softball—the list is endless. Raise that heart rate and sweat a little. It's great for the mind and the body.

You need to find an activity that feels right for you. Some people like the idea of joining a local health club, where there is an assortment of things to do, whether swimming, cycling, weightlifting, or running. Others prefer to work out in the privacy of their home. Some may like a competitive team sport outdoors, whereas others may prefer a solo activity indoors. When taking up a physical activity, go with what interests you and see if you enjoy it. If you don't, look for something else until you find an activity that is right for you.

You should also exercise for health reasons, but be sure to check with your doctor before you begin any exercise program. Your drinking may have taken more of a toll on you physically than you realize. You don't want to compound any problems by starting out too fast.

Aerobic Exercise Releases Endorphins

Aerobic exercise refers to any sustained activity that uses large muscle groups. Active muscles consume oxygen, so the lungs and heart must work harder to supply it than when a body is at rest. Examples of aerobic exercise are jogging, bicycle riding, brisk walking, stair climbing, or swimming.

Aerobic exercise releases chemicals called *endorphins* in the body that are involved in fighting pain and emotional stress. Endorphins put you in a state of relaxation and give you a positive outlook. Endorphins can also be released through meditation.

Set Realistic Exercise Goals

Start slow. You don't want any injuries or setbacks, and you certainly don't want to discourage yourself by setting unrealistic goals. Don't begin by setting a goal of exercising five times per week for one hour each day. Instead, start off by taking a 10-minute walk a few times each week. As you feel more inclined, you can begin to do more. Even if you are badly out of shape, if you start slowly, you will eventually build up stamina and strength. But don't forget to see your doctor before starting any exercise program.

CHANGE YOUR LIFESTYLE

As you can now see, if you are going to succeed in your effort to stop drinking, you must change your lifestyle significantly so that drinking, once your favorite leisure activity, is replaced by other healthier (and more fun) activities. In addition, many of the things you liked to do while under the influence of alcohol you will now have to enjoy without it: card games, barbecues, golf, softball games, bowling, seeing certain friends, fishing, or even watching TV. It's quite an adjustment but entirely possible. For instance, Rob began to play golf with his father instead of playing golf with his drinking friends, and he learned to enjoy it even more sober than he had golfing and drinking with his friends. Jim started to go fishing with his wife rather than going by himself and consuming too much beer.

Keeping busy and learning to structure your day with alcohol-free activities is the best way to start, as this prevents boredom, keeps you busy, and keeps you from thinking about drinking. Over time, scheduling and doing these activities will become automatic and a part of the new, nondrinking you. When you put your mind to it, there are many things that you can do. Enjoyable activities will strengthen your commitment to not drinking because your new life will be so satisfying and rewarding that you will not want to lose your new-found benefits.

Look around—you may also find new pleasure in things you've overlooked that were already a part of your life. For example,

—John discovered that he loved to watch his boys play hockey and eventually got involved in coaching;

—Bill developed a passion for lawn care and spent hours keeping up his yard; and

—Margaret found that she loved to experiment by cooking fancy new meals.

DEVELOP HEALTHY PEOPLE CONNECTIONS

It is important to have people in your life who care about you and support your effort to achieve abstinence. It's just as important not to associate with people who will jeopardize your lifestyle change. This means that you may need to make new friends and stop associating with some old ones. When you drank, chances are you associated with others who also drank heavily. These drinking friends may even have alcohol problems themselves. As a part of your lifestyle change, you may no longer be able to see and do things with your "drinking friends."

Continuing to See Your Drinking Friends Is Dangerous

Let's face it. It will be extremely difficult, if not impossible, for you to continue to associate with your drinking friends and remain abstinent. Remember what I said earlier (chapter 11) about making the commitment to abstinence. As important as old friends are, if abstinence is your number one priority, you need friends who do not have alcohol as their top priority either.

In the unlikely circumstance that you continue to see your drinking friends without it affecting your abstinence, you may no longer enjoy seeing them anyway. You won't have drinking in common. It is boring to sit around and watch everyone else get drunk, and you'll learn that it's impossible to have a meaningful conversation with someone who is drunk. Even fun activities aren't much fun when everyone is getting intoxicated. You'll also see how silly and stupid your good friends act when drunk. Now that you are sober, stories and antics you once thought were funny will no longer seem so cute.

Admittedly, it is not easy to cut ties with your friends. You might talk to your friends about your decision to abstain. Perhaps you can agree to see each other only when alcohol is not present, at least until you are comfortable with your decision to change your lifestyle. Seeing your friends individually, as opposed to all together, might be an option, as long as the friends you see agree not to drink. If your friends cannot agree to do this, it says something about the power that drinking has over them.

Reconnect with Your Friends Who Don't Drink or Who Don't Drink Heavily

You may have some friends that you lost touch with because of your drinking lifestyle, friends who can take or leave alcohol. This is an excellent time to reconnect and reestablish friendships that were not based on your drinking together. Since drinking is not the mainstay activity for these people, you may be able to socialize with them without risking a return to drinking. You can even talk to them about your decision not to drink. They will in all likelihood support your decision and encourage you to stick with it.

Developing a New Support System Takes Time

It is not easy to develop a new support system of friends and acquaintances, especially if all of your friends are heavy drinkers. If this is the case, when you first stop drinking, you will feel very lonely and disconnected, like a fish out of water. Being isolated can lead some people to drink as much as associating with drinkers leads others to drink. This is a normal reaction, and you should anticipate it.

That is why, when developing your new lifestyle, you should get involved in group activities that you enjoy, as this will give you an opportunity to meet other people with interests similar to yours. Enrolling in a class or joining a hiking, biking, or conservation club are ways to meet people where drinking is not the common activity. As I mentioned earlier in this chapter, check out the app Meetup to find groups of people who share your interests.

Coping with feelings of isolation is another reason why many people find support groups such as Alcoholics Anonymous helpful. Attending meetings gives you an opportunity to meet new people who aren't into the drinking scene, cuts down on any feelings of isolation you may have, and helps you develop a new support system.

Without making a commitment to attend meetings forever, you may find attending them helpful in the short run.

A new way to meet other people who do **not** want to drink is to go to alcohol-free bars. These are venues that look and feel like bars, where you can meet people who like to socialize without drinking alcohol. Alcohol-free bars are fairly new but are growing in number. Going there could be another way for you to meet people who have no interest in drinking.

Try not to get frustrated. Remember that it takes time to make new friends and change old habits. Meeting new people and making new friendships will happen naturally in time if you keep busy, develop new interests, force yourself to explore nondrinking social opportunities, and continue to work at it.

Romance

While there are no hard-and-fast rules, it is wise to avoid starting a new romantic relationship until you feel secure in your abstinence from alcohol. A new love takes your focus off your drinking problem and can replace abstinence as your most important priority. In subtle ways, a romantic connection can take energy away from your commitment to stop drinking. You may even make some decisions for the sake of the new relationship instead of considering the outcome of those decisions for your commitment not to drink.

For example, your new love interest may want to go someplace where alcohol will be readily available. Although you know this is not the best situation for you to be in, rather than saying no, you might go anyway and end up drinking. Or perhaps your new lover drinks socially, and rather than refusing to drink and explaining why you don't, you join in and begin drinking again.

Additionally, the highs and lows of a romantic relationship can be significant factors in returning to drinking. If you enter into a new relationship that does not go well, the pain and difficulties can lead you to take that *one drink* in an effort to feel better. In short, romantic interests are complicated enough in the best of circumstances, and you do not need any added complications until you are secure in your new alcohol-free life.

I understand that it may be hard to avoid new love, so if you do enter into a romance, remain vigilant and keep your focus on where it belongs—not drinking. And before you seek a new relationship, give yourself enough time to feel secure with no longer drinking.

SUMMARY

There are so many things you can do to keep busy, pass the time, and not drink. Experiment and have fun trying new activities. Find interests you enjoy that will help you not drink. It may take some time for you to figure out what really interests you, but that's OK. There is no rush. Eventually, though, these activities will become a part of the new you who enjoys life even more without drinking.

Granted, it can take a while for these changes to occur, but there will be a time when you don't miss drinking, don't think much about it, and enjoy your new life even more than your former one. Use your imagination and immerse yourself in all that life has to offer. You'll never regret it.

CHAPTER 13

Managing Urges to Use

Subdue your appetites, my dears,
and you've conquered human nature.
CHARLES DICKENS

After quitting, you may experience intense urges to drink. Some people report that an urge can feel almost like a physical craving that strongly tempts you to drink. If you do suffer from this type of urge, it's important to know that an urge can come days, weeks, months, or even years after quitting, and may continue to come throughout your life. Typically, though, urges decrease in their intensity and frequency over time, and many people report that they go away. If you experience an intense urge, you should never give in to it. Urges are caused by a combination of biological, psychological, and environmental factors.

People who quit smoking crave nicotine in the same way, as do people who used to be dependent on drugs such as painkillers or cocaine. When a person habitually uses a substance, the person's brain gets used to having it. Long after the substance has been withdrawn, there are times when the brain remembers the positive feeling it once offered. You experience this as a craving. Particularly when something in your environment reminds you of drinking, your brain can be activated and cravings can begin. Abstinence can hinge on your skill at being able to resist these urges.

MAINTAIN YOUR ENERGY LEVEL

Combating an urge to drink takes good decision-making. Your "thinking brain"—responsible for controlling your behavior, reasoning things through, and taking into account any risks involved when you take action—must be sharp. When you and your thinking brain are tired, you don't think as clearly and exercise poorer judgment. You don't want to be in that position. To make sure that "all your brain cells are firing," you need to get a good night's sleep. When your energy level is up, your thinking brain is strong, which helps you combat any urges to drink.

Unfortunately, sleep difficulties are quite common for people who have just stopped drinking, and they can persist for months. Problems include falling asleep, staying asleep throughout the night, and waking up earlier than usual. The first thing to keep in mind is not to be alarmed by this, since it is a common problem. Remember, too, that as uncomfortable as this is, a better sleeping pattern will return with time.

To help you get a good night's sleep, avoid drinking any caffeinated beverages in the afternoon and evening because this will only make the problem worse. Also, try not to take naps during the day, and develop a regular time when you go to bed. Over time, doing these things will help you reestablish a better sleeping pattern.

In addition to trying to get a good night's sleep, also make sure that you aren't overdoing things and that you are getting the rest you need. Find balance in your life: if things are stressful for you and you feel drained, take time for yourself to rejuvenate, relax, and rest. Try meditating, take a bath, or take a leisurely walk; or just sit down, take some deep breaths, and, as you exhale slowly, say the word *relax* to yourself. Take a break from things when you need to in order to maintain an adequate energy level.

Finally, remember to eat well, too. This is something you probably never thought much about when you used to drink, but a proper diet also helps you maintain a good energy level and decision-making abilities. A combination of carbohydrates, protein, and fat is essential. If you need help knowing what to eat, speak with your doctor, who can refer you to a nutritionist.

Heavy drinking is associated with deficiencies in essential vitamins A, B, C, D, E, and K because alcohol inhibits their absorption. Deficiencies in the minerals calcium, magnesium, iron, and zinc are quite common as well. If you don't want to see a nutritionist, at least take a daily multivitamin.

WANTING TO DRINK IS NORMAL

Wanting to drink again is normal and to be expected, even when there is nothing particularly stressful going on in your life. It is highly likely (and not a sign that you are crazy) that despite all the problems it has caused you, you still desire alcohol. You like to drink, and much of your drinking was enjoyable. If you didn't like to drink, you would not be in this predicament, and like people with an addiction to another substance, you have a disposition to drink. This is why cravings might well pop up throughout your lifetime. So don't be surprised when you experience them. You need to accept that they are a part of staying abstinent, and you must develop ways to manage them.

TRIGGERS

A *trigger* is a social, environmental, or emotional cue that reminds you of drinking alcohol and can give you an urge to drink again. Even the thoughts you have can be a trigger and cause a craving to drink.

External Triggers
External triggers are people, places, and things that have become associated with your drinking. Even times of the day or times of the year can be a trigger. Being at a party, associating with certain people,

attending a sporting event, seeing a television commercial that advertises alcohol, walking by a bar where you used to drink, or even seeing an empty bottle of alcohol can be a trigger for you. Anything outside you that can give you a desire to drink is one of your external triggers.

You may notice that your urges come at certain times of the day or in particular situations. This is because your drinking was linked to particular events or parts of your daily routine. Think about it: you probably drank after work, on payday, at a sporting event, with particular friends, or when you were alone. Many people never think about alcohol when they are at work, but toward the end of the workday or when arriving home, alcohol comes to mind. The situations that elicit your urge to drink are your external triggers.

Internal Triggers
Internal triggers are often more subtle and can be puzzling. People may report that an urge to drink came up without their knowing what triggered it. But if you pay close attention to your mental state at the time, you may discover what produced it. Feeling happy, feeling worried about something in your life, missing alcohol, or experiencing physical pain can all be triggers. So too can minimizing the severity of your alcohol problem and thus thinking that you can have just one drink and maintain control. Thoughts and feelings that tempt you to drink are your internal triggers.

Discover What Triggers Your Urge to Drink
It is important that you get to know your triggers. Learning to identify your triggers means you can avoid those situations. If you cannot avoid your triggers, you can at least plan ahead to do something different when you experience one. Learning ways to cope with your triggers is key to success.

Let's say that much of your drinking occurred after work, and you notice that you begin to think about and crave alcohol as the end of the workday approaches. This means you need to change your routine of getting off work, going home, and making yourself a drink. Instead, vary your plans. Could you go home later? Stop at the supermarket on the way?

For instance, Joe used to get home about one hour before his wife, and he struggled not to drink during this time. He decided to speak with his boss about shifting his work hours so that he could work later and arrive home right after his wife. This change of schedule eased his struggle and took away his trigger. If payday triggers your urge to drink, ensure that you have plans in place for after work on payday that do not include drinking. Jim found that payday was a difficult time for him because all of his coworkers went to the local bar after work. He decided to go into work later that day so that he would have to stay later and wouldn't be available when everyone left to go drinking.

Aubrey struggled with her drinking for many years. Her history was to have cycles of abstinence followed by heavy drinking. She found that after being abstinent for a couple of months, she began to ruminate about drinking and crave alcohol. When she looked at this closely, she realized that after a period of not drinking, she started to minimize her drinking problem and to think there would be no harm in having just a couple of drinks. Inevitably for her, a couple of drinks led to heavy drinking once again. Thinking she could drink moderately was her internal trigger, and she learned to catch this thought. She forced herself to think of all the times when having two drinks had resulted in out-of-control drinking, and she stopped herself from believing that she could drink in control.

Paula struggled with chronic pain and realized that this was a trigger for her. Instead of drinking, she learned to cope with her pain through meditation and remembering that alcohol was not the answer.

PAY ATTENTION TO YOUR FEELINGS

Strong negative feelings such as anger, resentment, sadness, and stress can often trigger an urge to drink. While there is never any good reason to drink, you don't want to let these feelings build up inside you, or else you might convince yourself that you deserve a drink. Instead, you need to listen to and address your feelings.

On a daily basis, take the time to monitor how you feel and truly listen to yourself. Ask yourself if you're feeling bothered, upset, or stressed by anything. If you are, this is a sign that you need to change something in your life, and your goal is to figure out what you need to do in order to feel better.

Nicole, for example, had stopped drinking for six weeks and found herself feeling so upset that she started ruminating about drinking again. She came to realize that these feelings were due to some problems she was having with her boyfriend, so instead of sitting on these feelings (or drinking to numb them), she talked with him, which greatly improved their relationship and helped to take away her desire to drink.

Adam had a stressful job and used to drink to deal with his feelings. After he got sober, there were times when he continued to feel stressed, and it was during these times that he began to think more about drinking. However, instead of his usual pattern of trying to ignore these feelings and drinking, he spoke with his boss, who supported his request to get some assistance with his work. He also started to exercise after work as a way to relax.

Attending to your feelings and using them as a guide for action will feel new to you if you used to drink to cope with them. Doing this will take some practice, but it will be worth the effort. Some people may find it helpful to talk with a professional therapist as they learn to deal with their emotions, which is an option I cover in chapter 17.

Feelings Are Important, but So Are Your Thoughts

While feelings can trigger a craving for alcohol, feelings in and of themselves do not lead to drinking. Along with feelings, there is always a thought that is involved, which is *thinking that alcohol will take away the pain and make things better.* That thought is not always recognized, but it is there. In the moment, when dealing with an urge, people will tell themselves that alcohol will decrease their stress, take away their pain, or help them cope. Thinking that alcohol will help is always something to watch out for.

"MY TRIGGERS AND HOW TO HANDLE THEM" EXERCISE

At the end of this chapter, there is the worksheet My Triggers and How to Handle Them, which you should complete. Think of all your potential triggers that can bring on an urge to drink. These are all those people, places, and things as well as those internal thoughts and feelings that can give you an urge to drink. If you can avoid your triggers, great. If you cannot, then come up with some strategies to deal with them without drinking.

Alex realized that going to a sporting event was a trigger for him, and he made the decision not to go to any until he felt more confident in his sobriety. Maggie had a stressful job whose stresses she could not avoid, so after work she began to take long walks to unwind. Craig did much business travel, and being alone in the evenings in a hotel room was a trigger for him. He decided always to pack a good book to read, and he got into the habit of taking a warm bath to relax.

YOU DIDN'T QUIT BECAUSE YOU DISLIKED ALCOHOL

Remember that your decision to stop drinking had nothing to do with your no longer wanting to drink alcohol. Rather, you made the decision to quit because of all the problems your drinking had caused.

I stress this point because the reason that many people go back to drinking after a period of abstinence is simply because they want to. You, too, may encounter a time when you crave alcohol. If this happens to you, you can become confused about why you are not drinking, and you may choose to forget about your alcohol-related problems. Your thought process might go something like this: "I am dying for a drink . . . Why shouldn't I drink? . . . It will make me feel better . . . Why should I deny myself this pleasure? . . . After all, I have had a tough day (or a difficult week or month) . . . I deserve it."

Quash the urge. If you don't put a stop to this type of thinking, it is a sure bet that you will soon be drinking again. Instead, you must force yourself to remember the unpleasant ramifications and forget the pleasurable aspects of drinking.

URGES GO AWAY EVEN WITHOUT DRINKING

The good news is that *even an intense desire to drink passes.* I hear from people who say that, when they craved alcohol, they took their mind off it by doing something else, such as going for a walk, making a phone call, or baking cookies; and within a short time, like magic, the craving was gone. So, your goal must always be to get through the *temporary* urges to drink without drinking. An urge can be powerful like a wave, but if you ride it out, it will pass. The following are ways to get drinking off of your mind.

Don't Dwell on the Urge to Drink; Distract Yourself Instead
In truth, the more you think about drinking, the more likely you are to drink, especially when you are experiencing a powerful urge to drink. *Dwelling* means continuing to think about how nice it would be to have a drink. When you begin thinking this way, you give your mind the opportunity to convince yourself that it is okay to have a drink. So don't dwell! Instead, get involved in some other activity,

such as jogging, walking, showering, or talking to a friend. Perhaps you can go shopping or begin to read a book. Anything that can redirect your focus at the moment can help. Your goal is to get past the urge and through the moment without drinking.

Chuck found that heavy exercising helped him get past an intense urge to drink. He would go for a long jog, and by the time he got back home, he had lost the urge to drink. Bob would immerse himself in singing along to loud music. He would get so involved in this that he could not think about drinking, and the urge would eventually disappear. So find something that you enjoy, and do it whenever the urge strikes.

Break It Down into Small Units

Urges to drink do not last forever. They do pass, and it helps to remember that they are time limited. The way to get through them is tell yourself that you only need to not drink for five minutes. Put your energy into doing something different and distracting that does not include drinking for that small period of time. You may find after five minutes that the urge has gone away. If it hasn't, then tell yourself that you can do another five minutes, and so on, until it has passed. It is much easier to deal with urges by remembering that they will pass and by distracting yourself for short periods of time.

Think the Drink Through

"Thinking the drink through" means forcing yourself to imagine what will happen if you start drinking again. If you have trouble getting rid of an urge, slow things down and make yourself remember what will happen if you drink again. Here's how:

Focus on the Harmful Consequences. When you feel the urge to drink, remind yourself of your reasons for not drinking. Those ambivalent feelings about quitting that everyone has (see chapter 4) have an uncanny way of creeping back into your mind and can begin to take over. They may push out the positive aspects of not drinking, causing you to lose sight of the harm you caused yourself by drinking. To combat this, reread the list you've written of harmful consequences of your drinking, and focus on this instead of taking the first drink. You should carry this list around with you at all times for quick reference in case you experience an urge and start to forget. This would also be a good time to reread the goodbye letter to alcohol that you wrote. That letter was designed to keep fresh in your mind why you have made the decision to end your relationship with alcohol.

The Morning After. If you do give in, I guarantee that you will remember the negative consequences of your drinking *after* you take that drink. The next morning, for example, you will regret it and feel bad about doing it. Perhaps you will have a hangover or the recurrence of a problem caused by your drinking. I have never heard a person who drank again after a period of abstinence say, "That was a good decision. I'm glad I drank again."

No matter how you look at it, giving in to an urge to drink is a bad move and does not make your life any easier. Stay on the alcohol-free path, and do what you can do not to veer off it. In the long run, this will help you achieve your goal of sobriety.

Focus on What You Don't Want to Lose. Now that you've created a fulfilling life without alcohol, you should want to keep it that way. You have worked hard, and there are people and activities bringing you joy in life that you don't want to lose. Reminding yourself of this also helps combat urges to drink.

JUST BECAUSE YOU WANT TO DRINK DOESN'T MEAN YOU SHOULD—EVER!

I want to share one of my favorite mantras with you in the hope that you'll practice saying it to yourself: "Of course, I want to drink. However, I can choose not to because I don't want to deal with the consequences that have resulted and will result from my drinking." When you feel the desire to drink, repeat this. Over time, this mantra, along with the other advice in this chapter, should help you develop confidence that you can successfully handle urges.

Remember, too, that you have a choice between drinking and not drinking. For some, the idea that they *can't* ever drink again bothers them tremendously. To fight this, they tell themselves, "Who says I can't drink?" When they remember that they *can* drink but that they *choose* not to, they feel comforted. Of course, you can drink again if you want to drink. You simply are choosing not to do so on that day because your life is better when you don't consume alcohol.

REACH OUT FOR SUPPORT

It can be particularly helpful to talk about your intense urge with someone who knows you are trying to stop and with whom you feel comfortable. This person should also be available when you need to talk. This person may be your partner, spouse, sibling, parent, or friend. It doesn't matter. What does matter is the person's willingness to help and your respect for that person's opinion of you.

Scott discovered that whenever he felt like drinking, calling his wife, Sandy, and talking with her about how he was feeling always helped him get past his urge. "After I speak with her and tell her that I won't drink, I just can't," Scott said. "I don't know if it's that I can't let her down or me down, but the decision is made, and then I just do something else until I see her. And once I see her, I know the battle is over."

Making the effort to talk with someone about your urge to drink often can take the urge away. Make sure this person can remind you of the reasons why you are not drinking, which you will need to hear to overcome your urge to drink.

SUMMARY

Overcoming the urge to drink is an important skill and one you'll need to master so that you can quit drinking successfully. The good news is that there are many ways to handle urges and remain sober. And believe me, over time you will get better and better at doing this, and urges will come less often and will usually be less intense. Remembering the following will help you handle your urges:

- Wanting to drink is normal and to be expected.

- Urges can and do go away without drinking.

- Figure out what your triggers are and avoid them, or make changes in your life to handle them.

- Distract yourself and don't dwell on the urge.

- Get through urges five minutes at a time.

- Think through the urge by focusing on the negative consequences of drinking and what you will lose if you drink.

- Remember that there will always be times when you want to drink and that you can choose not to drink.

- Reach out for support.

My Triggers and How to Handle Them

My trigger	Can I avoid it? yes or no If no, what can I do to handle it?

CHAPTER 14

Slips and Falls on the Path to Sobriety

Just keep going. Everybody gets better if they keep at it.
TED WILLIAMS

A person who is trying to stay abstinent, especially a newly sober person, will often slip (lapse) or fall (relapse). A slip or lapse is when a person temporarily returns to drinking for a short period of time and doesn't suffer major consequences as a result. A fall or relapse is a heavy involvement with alcohol after a period of abstinence that likely comes with bigger alcohol-related problems. When trying to stay abstinent, any drinking is a serious matter, signaling that you are not in control and that trouble is just around the corner. Obviously, the more lapses you have, the greater the chance you will eventually have a relapse.

When you first stop drinking and achieve some success in abstinence, you can grow confident, even cocky, and the structure and careful decision-making that enabled you to stop drinking can erode. For example, you may resume activities you previously avoided where alcohol is available, or you may begin to reconnect with friends who drink heavily. You might think you can handle these situations but then find yourself drinking again within a fairly short time.

To succeed, you need to maintain your focus on not drinking. Especially in the early months, you can't allow overconfidence to get in the way. You need to remember that, for you, drinking is an overlearned behavior. Not only must you learn and incorporate new skills, but you must also unlearn those deeply embedded, destructive old ones. Just like with learning a new golf or baseball swing, it is so easy to fall back to your old one. You have likely drunk for many years, and you probably cannot count all of the times you drank. Don't let down your guard. Staying sober still needs to be your top priority.

In this chapter, I discuss the three most common traps that will challenge your sobriety after a period of abstinence. Knowing about them can prevent a lapse or relapse. If you do lapse or relapse, this chapter will also help you understand what happened so that you can be on guard for it in the future. But first, let me say a few words about managing a lapse or relapse if it occurs.

MANAGING LAPSES AND RELAPSES

A lapse in not drinking is a real concern, but it does not have to result in a serious relapse. The quicker you end your lapse, the less harm it will cause to your future sobriety. If you have a lapse or even a relapse, minimize the harm. If you take a drink, it doesn't need to escalate into a relapse. For instance, if you take a drink, rather than saying, "Well, there's nothing I can do about it now, so I might as well get really drunk," instead say to yourself, "I drank, but I must stop now and prevent further harm to myself." Or let's assume you had a few drinks one evening. Instead of saying, "Well, I screwed up my sobriety, so I might as well drink tonight too," say, "Okay, I drank before, but I don't have to do it again."

Don't view a lapse or relapse as a personal failure, and don't beat yourself up over it. I always tell people I counsel that you can't change what happened in the past, but you can and should learn from it. A lapse or relapse can help you see where the holes are in your recovery program and what you need to work on to prevent a future slip. If you get really down on yourself for drinking again, your self-blame could lead to even more drinking. Finding fault with yourself does nothing positive for you and takes your attention away from your number one priority: abstinence.

Don't Discount Your Sobriety, but Don't Discount the Lapse

It is also important to remember that a lapse or relapse does not destroy your past period of abstinence and send you back to square one. If you were abstinent for two months and relapsed, or were abstinent for two years and relapsed, that is certainly better than drinking throughout this same time. Drinking again, while a serious concern, does not mean that you restart at the beginning. Feel positive about having been abstinent for that period of time.

On the other hand, don't minimize what has happened. You need to take seriously your drinking again. You need to understand what played a role in your return to drinking so that you will know what you need to do differently to achieve success.

Learn, Learn, Learn

If you return to drinking, think about what circumstances and events in your life precipitated your lapse. Life moves quickly, and we're often too busy to look closely at the factors that played a role in our decision-making. But this is exactly what you need to do to understand yourself better.

Try thinking of your life as a movie. Slow the movie down and look at it frame by frame. In one frame, you may not be thinking about drinking. In the next, you may have begun to think about it or actually started drinking. Review that micro-moment in extreme detail to see what was happening in your life and within your mind. Were you bored or lonely? Were you with people who were triggers for you, or were you in a drinking situation that was risky? Perhaps you were feeling particularly stressed. Closely examine what you were thinking and feeling and how you convinced yourself to drink again. By looking back in detail, you can learn what precipitated your slip and what you need to do differently to prevent this from happening again.

For instance, Dave, a 52-year-old man, had stopped drinking successfully for about four months. To his dismay, he found himself drinking again, which again caused him problems. He couldn't understand why he started drinking again, as his life had been going so much better since he had decided to stop. When he examined the circumstances of his relapse, he discovered that being away on business alone was the trigger. He realized that when he was alone at night with nothing to do, he began to ruminate about drinking, and eventually he began to drink. During those times, he had convinced himself that "no one would know anyway" and that, if he drank away from home, it "didn't really matter."

As a way to cope better with this situation, Dave learned to carefully structure his evenings when away on business and to plan activities after work that did not include being around alcohol. He also learned not to allow his thinking to trick him into believing that it was fine to drink when away from home. This insight and change in his behavior enabled him to avoid drinking in these situations, and he achieved abstinence again.

Like any new activity or endeavor, be it playing tennis, skiing, working on a computer, or golfing, refraining from drinking depends on learning and developing skills. Basic skills come first, and then, over time, more refined skills are acquired. As we practice, we get better and better at whatever task we are doing, including the task of not drinking.

If you drink again, the important point is to learn from the experience and to discover what you need to do differently so as not to drink in the future. The key is to learn from your mistakes so that you don't repeat the same ones over and over again.

THE THREE COMMON TRAPS

For more than 25 years, I have worked with people who struggle with their use of alcohol, and I've learned a lot about how people convince themselves to pick up a drink after having made the decision no longer to do this. Sometimes it happens because they simply didn't foresee a potential problem. They ended up in a situation where everyone was drinking, and before they knew it, they were drinking too. More often, though, it has to do with other factors. Amazingly, they often know these things, but at the moment they "forget" and don't think about them.

In the last three chapters, I reviewed a number of techniques and strategies you need to incorporate into your daily life so that you can achieve abstinence. I consider them to be the basics and essential for you to practice and remember. Although you have read about them, you, too, may "forget" about some of them, which can cause you to lapse or relapse. You also may not have fully integrated some of these strategies into your behavior, and this can contribute to your returning to drinking. So I will review some of those ideas for you now. There is a big difference between being exposed to skills and mastering them. The goal here is to re-expose you to some of these critical skills so that you can achieve mastery of them.

You need to be on guard for three main traps if you are going to stay on the path of sobriety. Knowing these traps will help prevent your returning to drinking and shed light on what is responsible for your setback if you have one.

1. Wanting to Drink and "Forgetting" the Consequences

Let's face it—you like the feeling of intoxication, and this led to your problem of drinking excessively. When you finally decided to stop drinking, the reason wasn't because you suddenly disliked alcohol but because drinking too much was causing you problems. You were sick and tired of the social, financial, legal, health, and other problems brought on by consuming too much alcohol. You may also have been fed up with how your use of alcohol was interfering with your ability to achieve your life goals. Your fondness for the feeling of intoxication, however, is a reason why it's difficult to follow a path of sobriety. That feeling of being high is hard to give up and often comes back to haunt you.

As I reviewed in the last chapter, there are going to be times when you'll crave a drink. I offered many ways for you to deal with this feeling, whether by not dwelling on it and pushing it out of your mind, distracting yourself, telling yourself to stay sober for short periods of time, or thinking the desire through and remembering the harmful consequences of your drinking. Despite knowing these techniques, many people return to alcohol simply because they *want to drink.*

Related to simply wanting to drink, people often tell themselves that they just don't care. They want to drink, and they convince themselves at the moment that they don't care what happens. *They simply want to drink.*

In past research of mine, I developed a questionnaire for people struggling with alcohol use that asked them whether they had ever relapsed and, if so, what had been responsible for it. The questionnaire offered about 35 different reasons for relapse, and people selected the most important ones. Of all the reasons they selected, one of the most common was *wanting to drink.*

If you've had a lapse or relapse and wanting to drink was a factor in it, go back and reread chapter 13 on how to manage urges to drink. Learning to resist a desire to drink and getting past that momentary feeling is critical. And let me again share with you one of my favorite mantras: "Of course, I want to drink. However, I can choose not to because I don't want to deal with the consequences that resulted and will result from my drinking." *You must force yourself to think the drink through and remember all of the harmful consequences that resulted from your drinking.*

Figure Out Why You Want to Drink. You should also consider why you want to drink so much. While the feeling of wanting to drink is normal for anyone who has had an alcohol problem, you may also experience a strong desire to drink because alcohol fills an important need you have. Is there something missing in your life now that alcohol is no longer there? If you can understand what alcohol fulfills for you, you can learn other ways to meet that need. Your desire to drink will then lessen, and you'll grow as a person.

Jerry was a 38-year-old single man who decided to abstain because he could no longer deal with hangovers and missing work. He stopped drinking for two months, but because of wanting to drink, he relapsed and started missing work again. Jerry began looking at himself to understand why he craved alcohol. He found that, without alcohol, he didn't know how to have a good time with others. Alcohol was his social lubricant and lessened his self-consciousness and anxiety. When he stopped drinking, he also stopped socializing and began to feel more and more isolated. Jerry began experimenting with alcohol-free social activities and forced himself to confront his anxiety. As he learned to have fun without drinking and to better manage his anxiety, his desire to drink decreased.

Understandably, this may be difficult for some of you to do on your own, especially if your anxiety is severe. In that case, you may need extra help to manage these feelings. Seeing a professional therapist, which I review in chapter 17, can enable you to develop the skills to do this.

As another example, Zach was a 32-year-old married man who stopped drinking after his use of alcohol had gotten out of control and was causing many fights with his wife. After not drinking for four months, he found himself ruminating about drinking and began to think that he wanted to drink, and he just didn't care what happened. When we looked closely at his thoughts, he was able to see that while he got along better with his wife without alcohol, he was not happy. He was not having any fun and was feeling bored with his life. Instead of drinking again, he spoke with his wife about exploring other recreational activities they could do together. They decided to go white-water rafting and hiking and made a plan to do some traveling together.

Try to discover why you like to drink so much. If you can, direct your efforts at satisfying those needs in other ways, which will decrease some of your strong urges to drink.

2. Believing You Can Control Your Drinking

Now wait a minute. How can the thought that you can control your drinking be responsible for a lapse or a relapse? After all, you may have already learned that you can't do this because you tried to moderate your drinking, weren't able to, and then chose to stop drinking entirely. Or you knew already that you couldn't learn to moderate your drinking, and without having to prove this to yourself, you decided on abstinence. In chapter 11, I reviewed the idea that abstinence is abstinence forever and that, for you, moderating drinking is impossible. How can you forget this, when forgetting allows you to decide to pick up a drink? Your mind has an amazing ability to forget the fact that you can't moderate your drinking. This forgetting is called denial. While you may have understood that you could not drink at all when you first began your path to sobriety, over time this thought often melts away and evaporates. What seemed so clear at the beginning becomes less so later on.

Denial. While, in the strict sense, denial refers to a person's failure to acknowledge even having an alcohol problem, in a broader context denial includes the minimization of a drinking problem, such as believing that one drink is acceptable. Acknowledging that alcohol is a problem but believing that it can be controlled, when it cannot, is also a form of denial. This form of denial sabotages sobriety and is a much more common variety than people believing they have no problem with alcohol at all. *People who struggle with alcohol have an amazing ability to overestimate their ability to control their use of alcohol.* You must guard against it.

Perhaps you have said one of the following things to yourself:

- "I have a problem, but I'm not that bad!"

- "Sure, I have an alcohol problem, but I can drink occasionally if I'm careful."

- "One drink won't hurt!"

- "I can control my drinking most of the time."

- "I haven't had a drink for two months, so I can have one or two drinks."

- "I can have one or two. I'll be fine!"

Sound like you? If you tell yourself that your problem isn't that bad, or that you can control your drinking after being abstinent so long, or that it is okay to have one drink if you're careful, you will eventually drink again. This same scenario occurs with other behaviors. Do you remember the slogan of the Lay's potato chip commercial: "Bet you can't eat just one"? Well, most people can't. One chip turns into too many. And the same thing happens with smokers or problem gamblers.

How often have you known friends who quit smoking and then, one day, decide to have a cigarette, *just one cigarette?* Before long, they are buying a pack. At the moment they had the first cigarette, they knew that cigarette smoking was a problem for them, but they convinced themselves that it would be fine to have just one. They never believed that having just one cigarette would lead them to full-blown smoking again. They denied the fact that they couldn't moderate their smoking.

Problematic Drinking May Not Happen Immediately. While there are some people who quickly lose control of their drinking once they begin to drink again, *even on that first occasion*, for many others, it is a slow and insidious process. They have a couple of drinks one evening, and nothing terrible happens, which persuades them that moderate drinking is possible. So, a week or two later, they drink again, which is followed by some drinking on the next weekend, and the next weekend, and then on a Thursday night. Over time, their drinking escalates, and they find themselves right back where they started.

The other danger of occasional drinking is that it can fuel urges to drink. While craving alcohol may have receded into the background after weeks or months of abstinence, "opening the door" by having some alcohol can reawaken urges for alcohol. This can lead to a struggle to maintain abstinence once again, if not to actual drinking. The bottom line is that you need to remember that drinking moderately is not possible.

Your Love of Drinking Causes Denial. The major factor that allows you to minimize your drinking problem is that you love to drink.

You don't want to admit that you can't drink at all because you enjoy drinking. So, in order to continue to drink, you tell yourself that your drinking isn't that bad or that you can control it.

In fact, if you didn't love drinking, denial would never be an issue. You would simply acknowledge that alcohol causes you problems, and you would stop drinking. After all, who wants to continue to do something that creates trouble? It is your love of alcohol and the wish to continue to drink that fuel the denial.

Overcoming Denial. Reread pages 165–166 in chapter 11. Those pages contain critical information that will help you avoid the trap of believing that you can moderate your drinking or even have one drink. Also review your written list of harmful consequences related to your drinking, as I suggested on page 163 of chapter 11. This will help you remember how bad your drinking really was and that you truly can't drink. You should also reread the cons of your drinking from the Pros and Cons of My Drinking exercise in chapter 4. Doing so will keep you alert to the seriousness of your drinking problem and what happens when you drink.

Finally, write down all of the times you unsuccessfully tried to limit your drinking and the times you planned to have just one drink (or a few) and, instead, drank to excess. I am sure there are many times you did this, and writing them down and forcing yourself to admit them counters the power of denial.

Thinking that your drinking can be safely controlled, and that one or two drinks will not lead to more, is an extremely common trap. *You must be on guard for this type of thinking.* Remember that this thinking is just your mind playing a trick on you. Knowing this will prevent you from falling for it.

3. Painful Feelings

Experiencing painful feelings is another big trigger that can lead you to break your sobriety and return to drinking. It is no wonder this happens. *Throughout your life, you have learned to use alcohol as a way to cope, and as a result, you never developed other, healthier ways to cope.*

For example, after having a stressful day at work, you would use alcohol to relax. After a conflict with a loved one, alcohol eased your stress. If you felt anxious or worried about something, alcohol was there. A relationship breaks up? Turn to alcohol. The easiest thing in the world is to find and justify a reason to drink.

When feeling upset, your customary way of coping was using alcohol. After years of doing this, your painful feelings and your use of alcohol got linked together. It is also true that, in the past, alcohol did help in some way. It took the stress away and provided some relief, at least in the short run. So now, when you experience any of these feelings, your brain remembers this, and your desire to drink increases.

In chapter 11, you learned that there is never a good reason to drink and that, regardless of what you feel, drinking isn't the answer. In fact, drinking will make everything worse, *which must be remembered in the moment as you can lose sight of that.* But when you feel pain, what can you do instead?

Sit with Your Feelings. First, learn to "sit with your feelings," and realize that you don't need to rid yourself of your painful feelings immediately. Learn to be more comfortable with feeling bad, which can be quite an adjustment for you. This is an important point because I bet you probably used alcohol as a quick fix to manage your discomfort. Whenever you felt bad, you drank, which at least temporarily took away your pain. Now that you aren't drinking, you aren't comfortable sitting with your feelings. Get to know your feelings, and don't be afraid of them.

Painful Feelings Get Better in Time. Understand that painful feelings often go away, or at least get better, within a fairly short period of time without your doing anything. What seems overwhelming at the moment often gets easier all on its own. You may not know this because you never gave yourself the opportunity to discover it. You drank, and if you felt better, you thought it was due to the alcohol. In reality, the alcohol may have had little, if anything, to do with it.

Take Mary, for instance. She used to get stressed at work and drank after work to cope. When she first stopped drinking, she was concerned about how she was going to deal with her stress. But what Mary found, much to her surprise, was that after a few hours, even if she didn't drink, she began to feel more relaxed. For her, it was an amazing insight.

Be patient. Sometimes it takes more than a few hours to feel better. You're not going to get over a relationship breakup overnight; however, you will get over it in time. Remember the one-day-at-a-time philosophy I reviewed in chapter 11. Just get through the day, which is all you need to do.

Try to Understand Your Feelings. Getting to know your feelings also gives you insight into yourself and what you need to do differently to feel better. For example, maybe you find that your pain consists of holding in the anger from a conflict you are having. If so, you need to express these feelings and face the conflict head on. If you find this difficult, there are books that can teach you how become more assertive and handle conflict. These can be found in most bookstores by looking for books with the word *assertiveness* in their titles. Or search for *assertiveness* at Amazon (www.amazon.com), where you can browse books on the subject. If managing anger is an issue for you, then search instead for *anger management*, and you will find books that can help you with that. You could also see a professional therapist for this kind of problem if you think you need extra help.

Some Techniques for Coping with Stress. If you are feeling stressed and worrying about something that could potentially happen that you have no control over, you need to remember to stay focused on the present and the day at hand and try not to worry about the future. Catastrophizing events in your day or imagining the worst will only make you more anxious. In fact, your worst fears may never come to pass, so it is good to deal with the future only when it arrives and not before. The Alcoholics Anonymous saying "one day at a time" can be extremely beneficial. In addition, it can be helpful to think about the positive things in your life and what you are grateful for. Remembering what you have and being thankful for it can bring you positive emotions that counter adversity.

It is also important to remember that while we may not be able to change a stressful situation or event, we can change how we view it. Without dismissing what has occurred, our perception of it can make all the difference. About the power of perception, William James, founder of American psychology, wrote, "The most amazing discovery of my generation is that a human being can alter his life by altering his attitudes." How we perceive and interpret a stressful circumstance will determine how much stress we feel. If you view it as a challenge as opposed to a crisis, you will keep your stress level lower.

Engaging in fun activities can also distract you from your concerns. While your concerns may not go away, you can at least get a temporary time-out from them. Always remember that there are other ways to manage things besides drinking. Deep breathing, walking, exercising, talking to a friend, or reading are ways to manage your feelings and get through a difficult time. Again, there are many books that can teach you techniques for managing stress in your life; these can be found in most bookstores or online at Amazon. The keywords to use in searching for books on this topic are *stress management*, *meditation*, and *relaxation training.*

Boredom and Loneliness. Common painful feelings in early recovery are boredom and loneliness, which can be uncomfortable and troubling. In fact, my research has shown that these feelings are some of the most common reasons for relapse. And it is no wonder that these feelings often trigger a return to drinking; after all, you are now trying to develop a new lifestyle, which may include finding new friends, a new support system, new interests, and new leisure activities. And developing a new lifestyle can be a frustrating process that takes time.

Chapter 12 explained how you need to change your lifestyle and fill the void left by alcohol. You don't want a lot of idle time on your hands, and you don't want to be a dry drunk. If you are experiencing loneliness and boredom, it is a sign that you need to put more emphasis on creating a fulfilling life for yourself without alcohol. Let your imagination loose, and come up with fun things to do.

SOMETIMES YOU MIGHT NEED HELP

There are people who, in addition to their alcohol problem, struggle with a psychiatric disorder, such as severe feelings of depression or anxiety. Others may suffer from a terrible self-concept, poor self-esteem, or have trouble developing meaningful relationships with others. If this describes you, know that there is help available, which I review in part V of this book. Remember that even in these situations, drinking isn't the answer. It will just make everything worse.

SUMMARY

In this chapter, you learned the three common traps that can knock you off track and lead you back to drinking:

1. Wanting to drink and forgetting the consequences

2. Believing you can control your drinking

3. Experiencing painful feelings

While you know that these aren't reasons to drink (in fact, there are no good reasons to drink), these traps have an insidious way of ensnaring you. It's easy to get fooled, and you can "forget" why you stopped drinking in the first place. Remembering these common traps can stop you from picking up that first drink and thus decrease the chance of your drinking again. And if you do lapse or relapse, knowing these traps helps you understand what happened and how to avoid another lapse or relapse in the future.

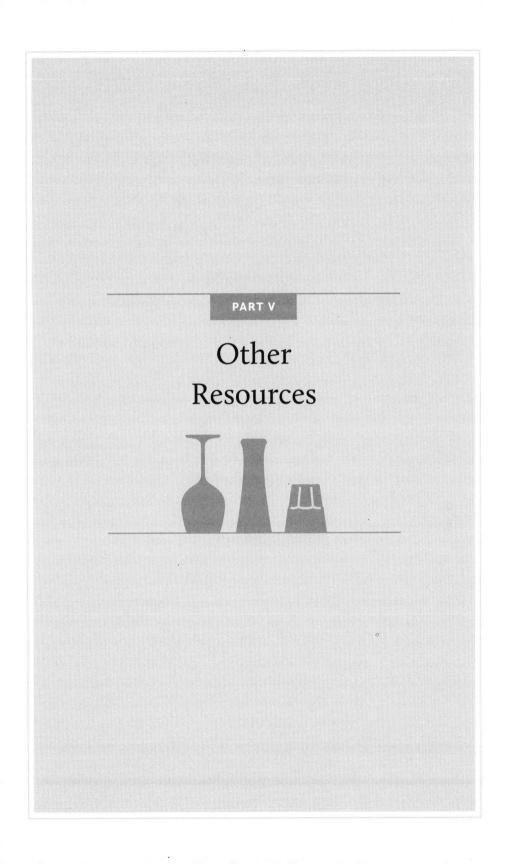

PART V

Other
Resources

CHAPTER 15

The Need for Outside Help

There is no failure except in no longer trying.
ELBERT HUBBARD

In spite of your best efforts and hard work, you may continue to experience problems related to drinking and may need to seek outside help. How do you know for sure if you fall into this category? If any of the statements below describes you, it is likely that you need help if you want to live a sober and happy life:

- You are not able to maintain abstinence for any significant period of time.

- You are able to achieve abstinence but occasionally relapse, with a return of drinking-related problems.

- You're unable to moderate your drinking and still will not consider abstinence, even though your life is full of alcohol-related difficulties.

- You have achieved abstinence, but you are not enjoying life.

- You have come to the conclusion that you need help to remain sober but aren't sure where to turn.

Any of these predicaments can be daunting or overwhelming. Whom do you turn to and where can you get the help that you need? You may have no idea what help is available and don't know where to begin. Or maybe you've heard of AA but aren't sure if it's for you, and you have no information about other kinds of help available.

On the other hand, you may have heard of many different kinds of treatment options—from hospitals, to rehabs, to outpatient programs, to halfway houses, to a range of self-help groups—but you don't know what's best for you, and you're confused about what to do next. Add to this all of the different types of therapists you may have heard of, such as psychologists, psychiatrists, social workers, and alcohol counselors, and your confusion can be magnified even further.

In today's world, with so many treatment options, you need to be an educated consumer. You want to get the right treatment the first time around rather than getting involved in the wrong program, or seeing the wrong therapist, and wasting your time. The good news is that choosing the best help is not as complicated as it sounds, and you can learn how to do it. But first, a few words about your decision to seek help.

DON'T BE UPSET WITH YOURSELF

You've tried hard to help yourself, and although you may have had some success, things still aren't where you want them. You may be thinking, "What is wrong with me?" or "Why can't I get it?" You may feel like a failure for being unable to help yourself with your problem, and that's a terrible place to be.

Try not to beat yourself up just because you need some additional support. Finding yourself a little stuck at times is human nature. The problem with getting a handle on your drinking may have absolutely nothing to do with your individual effort or the lack of it; difficulties occur for reasons that aren't in your control. In many cases, an outside observer can help you look at your situation in a different way, and with a new perspective, you'll succeed by trying a different route. Who cares if you need some help? The most important thing is that you're trying to help yourself and you're not giving up.

Don't let shame or embarrassment get in the way either. These feelings can stop you from getting the help you need. Even if you make it to your first appointment, they can get in the way of your being totally honest. You have nothing to be embarrassed about. You have a drinking problem, and that's it. Think back to chapter 2, when you learned why you may have a drinking problem. It has nothing to do with your character. You're just stuck in a certain way of being in the world, like we all get at some point in our lives.

SEEKING OUTSIDE HELP IS A POSITIVE MOVE

Taking control of your drinking problem is what this book is all about. Whether you're able to do this without any help other than reading this book, or you need some outside assistance, the important thing is that you are addressing your problem with alcohol. Your willingness to seek help demonstrates your commitment to getting better. That's something to be proud of.

In the next three chapters, you'll learn about the various types of outside help available to you. Almost all of these options maintain that abstinence is the only way to recover from a drinking problem. The only exceptions are the Moderation Management self-help program and meeting with a therapist privately and having moderate drinking as your goal for treatment. There may also be some professional therapy groups that have this as a treatment goal as well.

You'll discover that some of the formal treatment programs I review are highly structured and are indicated if you have been having a lot of difficulty resolving your drinking problem—for example, if you have not been able to put together any significant periods of sobriety and your drinking is still causing you major problems. Others are less structured and are more appropriate if you have been able to achieve some success but still have problems caused by your drinking. If you find that less structured treatment isn't helping you, you'll need more intensive treatment. If you continue to experience problems with alcohol consumption, even with treatment, abstinence *must* be your route to recovery.

SUMMARY

While some people can resolve their drinking problem on their own or by reading this book, others may need extra support and assistance. Despite their best efforts, these individuals continue to struggle with alcohol and are unable to resolve their drinking problem on their own. Or perhaps they want some outside support to make the process of getting better easier.

Do not be ashamed if you find that your own effort is not successful or that you want extra help. As I said previously, as with most any illness, alcohol problems run along a continuum, from mild to severe, and different types of intervention may be required to resolve the problem. Everyone is different, and what works to make a life change varies from person to person.

Acknowledging the need for outside help or wanting it is a positive decision. You are addressing your problem and not giving up, and that is the most important thing. What follows in the next three chapters is a description of the treatment options available, along with my advice about which ones may be appropriate for you.

CHAPTER 16

Self-Help Groups and Apps

Man is a social animal.

BARUCH SPINOZA

Self-help groups are outside the formalized, professional alcoholism-treatment system. In fact, self-help groups have been developed by people who struggled with drinking and were not getting the help they needed from professional treatment. In addition, these programs are free.

The first self-help program designed to help those who struggle with alcohol was Alcoholics Anonymous, or AA. Other self-help programs have been developed for the same purpose. These other programs were started because different things work for different people, and AA wasn't working for some people. Some found that AA wasn't a good match for them because of philosophical differences in how the program understands and helps a person who has a drinking problem.

Many people find self-help groups invaluable. Because you are surrounded by people who also struggle with alcohol, self-help groups can provide you with a place where you are accepted for who you are. If you're feeling bad about yourself, this welcoming environment can help you feel better. And if your present situation is very bad, being around others who have "been there" and have "gotten through it" can be wonderful and can remind you that there is hope and that you, too, will get through it. Being around others who struggle with the same problem as you do can also help reduce the destructive me-against-the-world feeling that you might have, when you find first-hand that there are many, many people in your situation.

Self-help groups can also provide you with a new social support system, which can be critically important if most people in your life drink. Remember that if you are going to stop drinking, you can't continue to associate with your drinking friends and be surrounded by alcohol. In addition, if you have lost many significant relationships because of your drinking, you'll have the opportunity to develop new friendships, which can help make up for these losses and fill the social void you may feel. And you will meet people who don't, or are at least trying not to, drink.

Attending meetings can also give you something to do with your time. As I mentioned before, loneliness and boredom are often huge concerns, particularly when you first stop drinking. You'll feel like you have an awful lot of time on your hands. There may even be times when you simply don't know what to do with yourself. Knowing that you'll be attending a meeting structures your day, gives you something to do, and wards off boredom and loneliness.

The most prominent self-help groups in the United States are AA, Moderation Management (MM), Secular Organizations for Sobriety (SOS), SMART Recovery, Women for Sobriety (WFS), and Refuge Recovery. Except for MM, all of these programs maintain that you must achieve abstinence to resolve your drinking problem. I will also review Rational Recovery, which used to be a self-help group but is now a self-help resource. Rational Recovery also insists on abstinence.

All of these programs have their own philosophy and ways of offering help; the key is to find one that fits with your own belief system. For some, AA has been an absolute lifesaver and the essential ingredient in resolving their drinking problem. Others have found that the philosophy of AA rubbed them the wrong way. They could never connect to that program and found much more benefit from another program. When looking for a self-help program, listen to your feelings and make the choice that's right for you.

In what follows, you'll learn about each program and its philosophy and approach, and this information will point you in the right direction. However, I encourage you to shop around, as there is nothing like experiencing a meeting firsthand to know whether it's right for you.

In addition to self-help meetings, an assortment of smartphone apps have been created in recent years to help individuals who struggle with alcohol and other drug problems. These are also outside the professional treatment system, although in 2017 the first mobile app was approved by the Food and Drug Administration to treat substance use disorders. There are now dozens of apps, and they each offer tools to help individuals attain abstinence. After I review self-help programs, I give an overview of the features these apps offer. As with self-help meetings, I encourage you to check out different apps to see which ones could benefit you.

ALCOHOLICS ANONYMOUS

Almost everyone has heard of AA, which is the best-known self-help recovery program in the world. AA estimates that it has more than two million members worldwide, with about half of those living in the United States, and there are more than 100,000 AA groups. Since AA first came into existence, many other self-help groups have taken its model for helping people who suffer from different addictions, including Narcotics Anonymous, Cocaine Anonymous, Pills Anonymous, Gamblers Anonymous, Debtors Anonymous, and Overeaters Anonymous.

AA was first developed in 1935 by Bill W. and Dr. Bob, both of whom were alcoholics. They began talking to each other, which helped Dr. Bob stop drinking (Bill W. was already abstinent), and soon after, both men began working with other people who struggled with alcohol. A few groups where alcoholics talked with other alcoholics began to meet, and four years later, AA published its basic textbook, *Alcoholics Anonymous*, informally known as the Big Book.

The Program

AA encourages total abstinence from alcohol. It believes that alcoholism is a disease and that recovery is a lifelong process. When people speak at meetings, they always mention their first name and the fact that they are an alcoholic or addict. When you first start attending meetings, however, you don't have to introduce yourself this way if you don't feel comfortable with it. AA advises that recovery from an alcohol problem can only be accomplished "one day at a time" by following the Twelve Steps of AA, the first of which is to admit your powerlessness over alcohol. A strong emphasis is put on a "higher power," however you choose to understand this, which exists outside you and helps you refrain from drinking. While AA is not a religious organization, it has a strong spiritual component.

There are different types of AA meetings, including speaker meetings, discussion meetings, step meetings in which the Twelve Steps of AA are discussed, and meetings for beginners, which often meet before a larger meeting. Meetings can be open to anyone or open only to those who have a desire to stop drinking. There are also more specialized groups for women, men, young people, and gay people. Groups vary in size from just a few members to hundreds of members.

In speaker meetings, members who have maintained abstinence tell their story. Speakers talk about when they first used alcohol, when and how their alcohol use became destructive, and, finally, their own salvation through abstinence and their involvement in the program of AA. Other members identify with aspects of these stories, which provide a model for their own recovery. There are also speaker discussion meetings, where a discussion takes place after the speakers have told their stories.

Discussion meetings generally focus on a particular aspect of the recovery process. These can be open to anyone or "closed" (open only to those who have a desire to stop drinking). Discussion meetings provide members the opportunity to discuss different aspects and phases of their alcohol problem. Discussion meetings can be

The Twelve Steps of Alcoholics Anonymous

1. We admitted we were powerless over alcohol—that our lives had become unmanageable.

2. Came to believe that a power greater than ourselves could restore us to sanity.

3. Made a decision to turn our will and our lives over to the care of God *as we understood Him.*

4. Made a searching and fearless moral inventory of ourselves.

5. Admitted to God, to ourselves, and to another human being the exact nature of our wrongs.

6. Were entirely ready to have God remove all these defects of character.

7. Humbly asked Him to remove our shortcomings.

8. Made a list of all persons we had harmed, and became willing to make amends to them all.

9. Made direct amends to such people wherever possible, except when to do so would injure them or others.

10. Continued to take personal inventory and when we were wrong promptly admitted it.

11. Sought through prayer and meditation to improve our conscious contact with God *as we understood Him,* praying only for knowledge of His will for us and the power to carry that out.

12. Having had a spiritual awakening as a result of these steps, we tried to carry this message to alcoholics and to practice these principles in all our affairs.

particularly helpful to newer members, who can direct their questions to longer-standing members who have a wealth of personal experience. Beginners' meetings are specifically for those who are just beginning AA, who have been sober for a shorter period of time, or who are returning to the program after a lapse or relapse.

In step meetings, participants discuss particular steps of the program. The steps are a progressive series of admissions and actions, spiritual in nature, that, when made or taken, can rid the alcoholic of the obsession to drink and help that person become happy and fulfilled.

Another important aspect to the program is choosing a sponsor who is another AA member in solid recovery. AA recommends finding a sponsor of the same sex to decrease the chance of any emotional distractions. By providing guidance and support, a sponsor can be a key individual in your recovery. Often a sponsor is available to talk to you by telephone and can meet you at or take you to meetings.

At meetings, you may hear about the absolute devastation someone has experienced from drinking, and this could make you think that you aren't "bad enough" to go to AA. Don't worry. The philosophy of AA is to identify with what you can and to forget the rest, which is good advice. AA uses the expression "There but for the grace of God go I." This means that whatever you hear could possibly describe you, perhaps not in your current state but at some point in the future. There are certainly people who, at an earlier time in their lives, could not believe the damage that alcohol would eventually cause them. When they first attended AA meetings and heard others tell their stories, they told themselves those things would never happen to them. Years later, however, their lives were even worse. Don't allow the feeling that you're not as bad as others prevent you from getting help.

For some, attending AA meetings becomes a way of life, and AA eventually becomes an important part of their identity. They may continue to go to meetings for the rest of their lives, and they may even go on "commitments," when they volunteer to speak at other

AA meetings to help other alcoholics. In addition, they may decide to become a sponsor to help others who struggle with alcohol. For others, AA is a once or twice a week meeting that helps them, and that is all they need. Many people attend meetings often in the beginning, when they need more support to stay abstinent, and then less frequently, after they have been sober for many months or years. Others may stop attending AA as soon as they feel comfortable not drinking and believe they no longer need the support of AA. While AA suggests that AA should become a way of life, it is fine to use it in a way that feels right for you.

If you decide to go to AA and eventually want to stop going to meetings, someone may tell you that you are headed for a relapse. Certainly some people have dropped out of AA and relapsed, but others have remained sober. Everyone is different, and no one approach is right for all. While some may need to remain in AA long term to recover from their drinking problem, others may benefit from a more limited involvement in terms of their frequency of attendance, their commitment to AA, and the length of time they continue attending meetings.

Finding Out More

A good way to learn about AA is to attend meetings. Because AA has many meetings, you are almost sure to find one near where you live. Go to at least two or three per week for a couple of months. Don't be put off if you don't like your first meeting. Every meeting has its own character and size. Check out some different meetings until you find ones that make you feel comfortable. Remember that the mix of individuals is different in each group, and some groups will feel better to you than others.

It is also common to attend a meeting where you can completely relate to the discussion, but on another occasion the meeting does not have the same appeal. This is normal and to be expected. AA suggests that you should "identify with what you can and forget the rest." This means that when you go to meetings, take in the things you hear that resonate with you, and if there are things that you can't connect with, simply disregard them.

Another excellent way to learn about AA is to talk to someone who is in the program. He or she would probably be happy to bring you to a meeting. To find out where meetings are held, check your local telephone directory for a listing for Alcoholics Anonymous or call the main number at (212) 870-3400. The AA office can tell you where meetings are held in your area and can send you a meeting booklet. For more information, write to AA at this address: Grand Central Station, Box 459, New York, NY 10163. A wealth of information is available at AA's website, www.aa.org. I would also suggest two of their publications: *Alcoholics Anonymous* (the Big Book) and *Twelve Steps and Twelve Traditions.* AA also has many online meetings. Information about those can be found at http://aa-intergroup.org.

MODERATION MANAGEMENT

MM was founded by Audrey Kishline in 1993, when she realized that there were no support groups for people who had problems with alcohol and wanted to try to moderate their drinking. She had struggled with drinking herself and received abstinence-oriented treatment, which she didn't find helpful. Over time, she began to moderate her drinking, and eventually she developed the MM program. The philosophy of MM is similar to my own presented in this book. It is the one self-help program that supports the goal of moderate drinking.

You may have heard that seven years after founding MM, Kishline killed two people in a car accident. She was intoxicated at the time, was arrested for drunk driving, and was sent to jail. At her trial, her lawyer said, "The accident and the subsequent intensive alcohol treatment she has undergone have made Kishline realize that moderation management is nothing but alcoholics covering up their problem."

I do not know the motive behind this statement, but some people who have struggled with alcohol are able to learn how to moderate their drinking so that alcohol no longer causes them problems. In chapter 7, I reviewed this concept and explained that some can learn to control their drinking while others cannot. Because Kishline could not learn to control her drinking does not mean that no one can succeed with this approach. In a similar vein, just because one person cannot learn to achieve abstinence does not mean that no one can.

The Program

MM is a behavioral-change support program for people who are concerned about their drinking. MM maintains that alcohol problems can vary from moderate to severe and that people should be free to choose their own goal for how to resolve their drinking problem, whether by abstinence or moderation. MM states that it is best for a person to address a drinking problem early, before it becomes more severe. MM also acknowledges that people who have serious alcohol problems will probably need to resolve their drinking problem by abstinence, but at the same time, MM maintains that such people need to figure this out for themselves.

MM offers nine steps toward moderation and positive lifestyle changes, and also gives recommendations about how much a person should drink.

Finding Out More

For more information about MM, you can call (212) 871-0974. MM's website, www.moderation.org, contains a lot of information about the program including where meetings are held. There aren't a lot of MM meetings, but MM maintains an active online community where members can get support. The book to read to learn more about MM is *Moderate Drinking: The Moderation Management Guide for People Who Want to Reduce Their Drinking* by Audrey Kishline.

MM's Nine Steps toward Moderation and Positive Lifestyle Changes

1. Attend meetings or online groups and learn about the program of Moderation Management.

2. Abstain from alcoholic beverages for 30 days and complete steps three through six during this time.

3. Examine how drinking has affected your life.

4. Write down your life priorities.

5. Take a look at how much, how often, and under what circumstances you had been drinking.

6. Learn the MM guidelines and limits for moderate drinking.

7. Set moderate drinking limits and start weekly "small steps" toward balance and moderation in other areas of your life.

8. Review your progress and update your goals.

9. Continue to make positive lifestyle changes and attend meetings whenever you need ongoing support or would like to help others.

Used with permission from https://www.moderation.org/meetings/readings.html, © Moderation Management Network Inc.

SECULAR ORGANIZATIONS FOR SOBRIETY

SOS, alternatively known as Save Our Selves, was formed in 1985 by Jim Christopher, who wrote an article about achieving sobriety through personal responsibility and self-reliance. After receiving an overwhelming response to this article, he eventually founded the organization.

The Program

SOS is a nonreligious support group for people who want to learn how to quit using alcohol or other drugs. It is an alternative to AA because it does not emphasize spiritual or religious beliefs. SOS believes that an alcohol problem is a separate, nonreligious issue. People don't need to be agnostic or atheist to attend. Anyone of any religious orientation is welcome. SOS emphasizes the importance of self-empowerment to achieve abstinence and asserts that no longer drinking must be the "Priority One, no matter what!"

SOS meetings usually are attended by about 12 people and are generally loose and informal. A chairperson often comes up with a topic to discuss, and everyone is encouraged to talk with one another about their experiences related to maintaining abstinence. Diversity and different opinions are respected, and there is an acceptance of each person's individuality and unique path into recovery. Although some may introduce themselves by acknowledging that they're an alcoholic or addict, this is not a requirement. Six guidelines are used to help people achieve their goal of abstinence.

SOS's Suggested Guidelines for Sobriety

To break the cycle of denial and achieve sobriety, we first acknowledge that we are alcoholics or addicts.

We reaffirm this truth daily and accept without reservation the fact that as clean and sober individuals, we cannot and do not drink or use, no matter what.

Since drinking or using is not an option for us, we take whatever steps are necessary to continue our Sobriety Priority lifelong.

A quality of life, "the good life," can be achieved. However, life is also filled with uncertainties. Therefore, we do not drink or use regardless of feelings, circumstances, or conflicts.

We share in confidence with each other our thoughts and feelings as sober, clean individuals.

Sobriety is our Priority, and we are each responsible for our lives and sobriety.

Source: James Christopher, *How to Stay Sober: Recovery without Religion* (Prometheus Books, 1988).

Finding Out More

To learn more about this program and where meetings are held, email SOS at sos@cfiwest.org or send a letter to this address: Secular Organizations for Sobriety, 2535 W. Temple Street, Los Angeles, CA 90026. The organization's website is sossobriety.org, which contains all kinds of information about the program. Jim Christopher has written three books about recovery without religion using the principles of SOS, and they can be purchased through the SOS Clearinghouse. If you can't find a physical SOS meeting where you live, there are dozens of online groups that use the principles of SOS.

SMART RECOVERY

SMART Recovery was developed in 1994 by a group of people who were originally connected to Rational Recovery. These people decided to develop a separate program because Rational Recovery moved away from its original principles. SMART Recovery has maintained its allegiance to the original ideas of Rational Recovery.

The Program

SMART Recovery is the second-largest self-help program for people with alcohol problems (the largest being AA). SMART Recovery doesn't view a problem with alcohol as a disease. It also does not use the concepts of a higher power or powerlessness, nor does it use the labels *alcoholic* or *addict*. It does, however, maintain that abstinence must be the route to recovery. SMART Recovery is obviously different from AA in its philosophy and orientation. However, it is perfectly fine for people to attend both SMART and AA meetings.

SMART Recovery teaches self-reliance rather than reliance on a higher power. It does not have sponsors. SMART Recovery understands addiction as complex, learned, and unhealthy behavior: a complicated bad habit. Because SMART Recovery holds that people have different needs and recover at different paces, it teaches that a person's need to attend meetings will vary, and no one has to attend meetings forever.

SMART Recovery uses scientific research and a "four-point program" in its meetings to help participants achieve abstinence. It helps individuals (1) enhance and maintain their motivation to abstain from using alcohol or drugs; (2) cope with urges and cravings to drink so that they don't have to act on them; (3) learn rational ways to manage their thoughts, feelings, and behaviors without using substances; and (4) balance momentary and enduring satisfactions.

SMART Recovery also uses the ABCs to help people overcome their addiction, teaching that when something happens—an "activating event"—this event leads to "beliefs, thoughts, or attitudes" that can be irrational or illogical. These lead in turn to "consequences" that are emotions and behaviors. By better managing one's beliefs and emotions that lead to drinking, a person can empower him- or herself to quit drinking.

Meetings are generally fairly small and are led by a "coordinator," who either is a person in recovery or is someone knowledgeable about the program but without a drinking problem.

Finding Out More

SMART Recovery has more than 300 groups both inside and outside the United States, and there are also many online meetings. You can contact the organization for meeting locations, recommended reading materials, and other information: 7537 Mentor Avenue, Suite 306, Mentor, OH 44060; telephone: (440) 951-5357. Its website is www .smartrecovery.org. Many books and publications about SMART Recovery can be found on the website. In particular, the *SMART Recovery Handbook* offers a thorough explanation of the program. Online SMART Recovery meetings can be found on the website.

WOMEN FOR SOBRIETY

WFS was founded by Jean Kirkpatrick, PhD, in the mid-1970s. Dr. Kirkpatrick struggled with drinking, and after she found that AA no longer helped her, she began to stop drinking on her own by changing the way she thought about her problems. She came to believe that, as a woman, she required treatment that focused on her self and self-confidence in addition to her alcohol problem. As she achieved success, she reached out to other women, which resulted in WFS.

The Program

WFS believes that heavy drinking is the way a woman learns to deal with emotional pain and that a part of recovery is learning healthier ways of dealing with painful feelings and problems. WFS teaches its members to replace negative, destructive thoughts with positive, self-affirming ones. In addition, its strong message is that all women are competent and can learn to be more self-reliant. In meetings, when a member introduces herself, she doesn't refer to herself as an *alcoholic* but rather as a *competent woman*.

Meetings provide a place where women can talk with and receive support and encouragement from each other. WFS suggests that meetings remain small, 6 to 10 people, so that everyone can have the opportunity to participate in the discussion on a topic related to drinking problems or something from WFS literature. Meetings are led by a member who has been abstinent for at least one year and knows the philosophy of the WFS program. WFS also maintains a pen-pal program so that members can communicate by mail or email when not in meetings.

WFS espouses the New Life Program, which has 13 "acceptance statements" for how members should deal with and think about life. WFS encourages members to take control of their lives through thought and action. It also maintains that abstinence is the only route to recovery.

WFS's New Life Program: Acceptance Statements

1. I have a life-threatening problem that once had me.

2. Negative thoughts destroy only myself.

3. Happiness is a habit that I will develop.

4. Problems bother me only to the degree that I permit them to.

5. I am what I think.

6. Life can be ordinary or it can be great.

7. Love can change the course of my world.

8. The fundamental object of life is emotional and spiritual growth.

9. The past is gone forever.

10. All love given returns.

11. Enthusiasm is my daily exercise.

12. I am a competent woman and have much to give life.

13. I am responsible for myself and for my actions.

© Women for Sobriety, Inc.

Finding Out More

For more information about WFS, contact WFS headquarters: Women for Sobriety, P.O. Box 618, Quakertown, PA 18951-0618; telephone: (215) 536-8026. The WFS website, www.womenforsobriety .org, contains a wealth of information about the program, including a list of many publications and books that can be purchased. You can find out where meetings are by checking out the website, by calling WFS, or by emailing WFS and saying where you live. WFS also offers an online community. Phone support is offered, as well as a message board and chat room. Two books to read about WFS, both written by Jean Kirkpatrick, are *Turnabout: New Help for Women Alcoholics* and *Goodbye Hangovers, Hello Life: Self-Help for Women*.

REFUGE RECOVERY

Refuge Recovery is a nonprofit organization grounded in the belief that the principles and practices of Buddhism can create a strong foundation to help someone achieve abstinence from a substance use disorder. It is a relatively new program, beginning around 2008. Refuge Recovery maintains that all have the power and ability to free themselves from the suffering caused by addiction. It believes that abstinence is essential for recovery.

The Program

Refuge Recovery thinks that people can train their hearts and minds to see clearly, and by responding to their life with understanding, they can free themselves from addiction. Refuge Recovery believes that the support of a community of peers is important. To accomplish this, Refuge Recovery is committed to building an extensive network of Refuge Recovery meetings and communities that offer Buddhist-inspired guidance and meditations for anyone seeking help for a substance use disorder. It recognizes Noah Levine, author of the book *Refuge Recovery*, as one of its founders.

Refuge Recovery maintains that there are four noble truths: addiction creates suffering; the cause of addiction is repetitive craving; recovery is possible; and the path to recovery is available. It also utilizes the eightfold path of recovery that consists of the following: understanding, intention, communication/community, action, livelihood/service, effort, mindfulness/meditation, action, and concentration/meditation. Its guiding principles consist of the following:

1. The group's health and well-being is of utmost importance.

2. Each group's core intention is to welcome and support those who are seeking recovery.

3. Groups are to be peer-led.

4. Refuge Recovery is an abstinence-based program.

5. Each group operates independently, except in matters affecting other groups or Refuge Recovery as a whole.

6. There are no fees for Refuge Recovery membership.

7. Ethical conduct can and should be practiced on a group level.

8. Our core principles are mindfulness, compassion, forgiveness, and generosity.

Meetings generally begin with a short introduction to Refuge Recovery, along with a reading of the four noble truths and the eightfold path. This is followed by a 20-minute group meditation. No one is expected to identify as an addict or alcoholic, and you don't have to be Buddhist to attend. After the meditation, the leader introduces a reading, or someone speaks about some other topic relevant to recovery, which is followed by an open discussion.

Finding Out More
More information about Refuge Recovery can be found on its website at https://refugerecovery.org. You can also contact the organization with any questions via email: refugerecoveryworldservices@gmail.com. The website contains a lot of information about the program and its practices and beliefs. The website also lists where and when meetings are held throughout the United States and offers meditation exercises that can be downloaded, as well as podcasts you can listen to. The book to read to learn more is *Refuge Recovery* by Noah Levine.

RATIONAL RECOVERY

Rational Recovery is included in this chapter because, at one point, Rational Recovery was a self-help group. Rational Recovery, however, changed its direction and is no longer a self-help group but is a self-help resource instead. Rational Recovery was started in the late 1980s by Jack Trimpey and used a type of therapy called rational emotive therapy to help people with alcohol problems. Rational emotive therapy is an action-oriented therapy that teaches people to examine their own thoughts, beliefs, and behaviors and replace self-defeating ones with more productive alternatives. In the early 1990s, the focus of Rational Recovery shifted to its present form.

The Program

Rational Recovery calls itself the antithesis and archrival of AA. Rational Recovery avoids the beliefs of powerlessness and a higher power. It also does not see an addiction to alcohol as a disease, nor does it believe that people need to be "in recovery" from their addiction to alcohol for the rest of their lives. RR maintains that people can completely recover and put their alcohol addiction behind them. The only thing RR and AA agree on is that abstinence is essential to controlling an alcohol problem.

When Rational Recovery was originally developed, it held meetings and used the ideas of rational emotive therapy. However, within a few years, Rational Recovery shifted its philosophy and now uses AVRT, or addictive voice recognition technique. Furthermore, the leaders of Rational Recovery began to believe that there was no need to go to meetings, so meetings were abolished. Thus, Rational Recovery is no longer one of the self-help meeting organizations. People achieve abstinence by visiting RR's website or by reading RR literature. By using AVRT, people learn to disregard their "addictive voice"—the thoughts and feelings that support their addiction. Users of AVRT are taught to recognize and take control of their addictive voice. Recovery is an event, and abstinence can eventually become effortless.

Recently, Rational Recovery has gone even further and now states that going to meetings or seeking any type of professional help impairs recovery because it takes away from personal responsibility. This thinking is incorporated into the organization's DPI, or Declaration of Personal Independence, which those interested should live by: "I will never, ever, attend another meeting of Alcoholics Anonymous or any other recovery group organization, nor will I obtain professional services of any kind, for the purpose of ending my addiction." Rational Recovery believes that the way to beat an addiction is through traditional values of individual responsibility, resiliency, self-reliance, and personal independence. From my perspective, Rational Recovery has taken things too far. While individual responsibility is important, there clearly is a place for professional treatment and self-help groups to assist people who struggle with their alcohol use.

Finding Out More

You can find out more about Rational Recovery by visiting its website at www.rational.org. The organization's contact information is as follows: Rational Recovery Systems, P.O. Box 800, Lotus, CA 95651; telephone: (530) 621-2667; email: rr@rational.org. The book that explains the organization's approach is *Rational Recovery: The New Cure for Substance Addiction* by Jack Trimpey.

SMARTPHONE APPS

Thanks to new technology, another option that might benefit you is a smartphone app (short for *application*). There are smartphone apps now for almost anything: improving your exercise routine or your sleep pattern, helping you lose weight or quit smoking or cope with depression or anxiety, or assisting you with learning a foreign language. There are also many apps designed to help you with an alcohol or other substance use problem. An app called ReSet by Pear Therapeutics has been approved by the Food and Drug Administration, but others have not attained this recognition and so fall outside formal professional treatment. That said, you still might find them to be helpful.

These apps offer a variety of features that may include reading or listening to information about alcohol use to attune you to your triggers and patterns of relapse and then completing a writing assignment. An app may offer daily inspirational quotations to keep you focused and motivated; a daily tracking of your mood and possible cravings; appointment reminders; text, audio, and video problem-solving modules; tools for coping with cravings; or tips for dealing with high-risk situations. Some offer a discussion board so that you can interact remotely with other people who are using the app.

Other apps have incorporated a proven method to help people who struggle with substance use called contingency management, which rewards people monetarily for attending any scheduled treatment appointment and for submitting random alcohol and drug test results. Tests can be done in privacy using a breathalyzer and oral saliva test, which are recorded in a selfie video and uploaded to a digital platform where they get reviewed. For additional support, some apps even offer a recovery coach who is typically an individual in recovery who can provide telephone or video chat support to the subscriber. Apps with these more sophisticated features can be downloaded for a fee, whereas others with fewer features are often available for free.

You can find these apps at Google Play if you have an Android phone or at App Store if you use an iPhone. Just type in *substance abuse*, *alcohol*, or *addiction*, and an assortment of apps will come up. Reading reviews should help you make a decision on what app to try.

SUMMARY

Outside formal professional treatment, there are many self-help programs that have helped millions of people. These include Alcoholics Anonymous, Moderation Management, Secular Organizations for Sobriety, SMART Recovery, Women for Sobriety, and Refuge Recovery. While different from each other, they all focus on attaining abstinence from alcohol (except for Moderation Management, which is designed to help a person moderate alcohol consumption). There are also many smartphone apps developed to help people address their drinking problem. These, too, vary in the features they offer.

If you find that you continue to struggle with resolving your drinking problem on your own or by reading this book, yet still don't want to get into formal professional treatment, you should consider checking out one or more of the self-help programs or apps. You may need to try more than one to find something that suits you. You may find this extra support to be exactly what you need to stay focused, manage your urges to drink, and keep motivated. Even if you are doing well, you may want to check out these self-help programs and apps, as you may find that you welcome the support.

CHAPTER 17

Professional Treatment

Never give in! Never give in! Never. Never. Never. Never.
WINSTON CHURCHILL

In addition to self-help groups, a whole system of professional care exists for you. Because different people require different types of care, a range of programs have been developed so that a person's specific needs can be met. Navigating this system can be confusing, as it's hard to know what kind of program you need, what kind of therapist to see, or even what's available. In this chapter, you'll learn about getting the care that's right for you.

You should know that the programs I review, in almost all cases, work with people who have an alcohol problem as well as those who have a drug problem or a combination of both alcohol and drugs. Therapists who specialize in the treatment of alcohol problems also usually specialize in the treatment of drug problems. I mention this because, if you get involved in any of these programs, you should expect to find some people there who struggle with drugs as opposed to alcohol. This, however, does not mean that these programs are not suitable for you. It is just that the professional treatment system is designed to work with people who struggle with substances, regardless of what the particular substance is.

INDIVIDUAL PSYCHOTHERAPY

Individual psychotherapy is a common choice for people who want help with their drinking. Some people prefer to speak to a therapist one to one instead of going to a self-help meeting. Others may wish to speak with a therapist in addition to attending some kind of self-help meeting because they have some concerns they want to discuss privately with a trained professional. You may find that your mood does not improve after staying sober, so you decide to speak with a professional to find out why you feel so bad. Psychotherapy can also be useful if you've been struggling to moderate your drinking and still want to see if you can learn to do so with some outside support.

Why Individual Therapy?

Individual therapy gives you the opportunity to look closely at yourself in a private way. Within an individual psychotherapeutic relationship, you and your therapist can explore what has prevented you from resolving your alcohol problem and what you need to do to accomplish that goal. Together, you will identify stumbling blocks and ways to overcome them.

Individual therapy can also be particularly useful if, despite abstinence, you feel awful. Whether the painful feelings were always there and you used alcohol, at least in part, to cope with them, or whether the feelings began after your drinking stopped, abstinence should not be a horrible, painful experience. Sure, some difficult times are to be expected, but abstinence should not feel terrible. Therapy can help you understand your feelings and move forward.

Choose the Right Therapist

When choosing a therapist, and prior to making an appointment, you should ask the therapist about his or her experience working with people who have alcohol problems. Don't be shy; this is critically important information. You should only see a therapist who has skill in working with problem drinkers. Even an excellent therapist, if he or she is not specifically trained in the treatment of alcohol problems, will not provide you with the help you need. Your health insurance company will be able to give you the names of some therapists who specialize in this area. Your insurer may also refer you to some substance use disorder programs that offer outpatient therapy. You can look online as well or possibly get a referral through one of your friends or your primary care physician.

Many different kinds of professionals offer individual psychotherapy. The list includes alcohol counselors; social workers; marriage, family, and child therapists; psychologists; and psychiatrists. Choosing the right one is important, so how do you decide? If the only issue you are dealing with is your alcohol problem, it's fine to see any of these therapists as long as they have the appropriate training in alcohol problems. However, if you have other concerns apart from your drinking problem, consider ones who have at least a master's degree or higher (licensed clinical social workers; marriage, family, and child therapists; psychologists; and psychiatrists) because these people generally have additional training for issues other than alcohol. You should know, though, that psychiatrists often don't see people for therapy but only prescribe medication, so if you call a psychiatrist, ask whether therapy is an option.

Whomever you see, within the first few sessions, you should feel that you can talk comfortably with your therapist and that this person can help you. If by the first or second session you find it hard to confide in your therapist or feel that the two of you just aren't connecting, you should shop around some more to find a therapist with whom you do feel comfortable.

There are also many, many different kinds of therapy. For example, behavior therapy emphasizes changing the behavioral patterns that cause you difficulties. In contrast, cognitive therapy focuses on identifying and correcting irrational and distorted beliefs that contribute to your distress. And cognitive-behavioral therapy incorporates features of behavioral and cognitive therapy by focusing on both destructive behaviors and negative thoughts. Finally, psychodynamic therapy explores your past to uncover what prior events may contribute to your beliefs, behaviors, and perceptions of the world that cause you problems. These are just four relatively common types of therapy; different therapeutic orientations number in the hundreds.

In my experience, therapists often incorporate features of different approaches to best meet the needs of their clients. Thus, I wouldn't be particularly concerned with the type of therapy the therapist practices. Again, focus on how well you connect with your therapist after a couple of sessions and whether you think this person can help you.

MARITAL AND FAMILY THERAPY

In marital and family therapy, you and members of your family meet together with a counselor to resolve problems, conflicts, and tension you have with one another. Even if you are already seeing a therapist individually, additional marital or family therapy may make sense if family problems are intense. In marital and family therapy, the focus isn't on you but rather on the relationships between family members. Sometimes even in individual therapy, one or more of your family members can be brought into a session to discuss a particular issue.

Whenever you plan to see a therapist for marital or family therapy, make sure that the person is skilled in this type of therapy. The nature of the work is much different from what occurs in individual therapy. Also make sure that the person knows about alcohol problems and how a family member's drinking can affect everyone in a family.

When you are involved in marital or family therapy, you should have your drinking under control or be abstinent. Continued problematic drinking should not be affecting your relationships with your spouse or other members of your family. Ongoing alcohol use can so complicate and confound what is going in a family that it is hard to know what the problems really are until alcohol is taken out of the picture. Continuing problematic drinking will exacerbate any difficulties you are experiencing and can also create problems that would go away if your drinking stopped. Simply put, marital and family therapy will not be effective as long as excessive drinking continues.

Why Marital or Family Therapy?
Drinking can cause a whole host of problems within your family, and even after you stop drinking, anger, resentment, mistrust, and other interpersonal problems can linger. People may not be talking to each other, and tension may be high. Marital or family therapy can help resolve those difficulties and get your family back on track.

GROUP THERAPY

Group therapy also can be helpful for the treatment of an alcohol problem. In groups, you can learn from others what has and has not worked for them, and you can get honest feedback from peers. Moreover, you will discover that you're not alone, that others struggle with alcohol, and that the support you can receive from other group members can be invaluable. Certainly, the self-help group programs reviewed in the last chapter offer these same features, which, at least in part, explain their success. If you don't feel comfortable attending a self-help group but still want a group experience, group therapy may be the answer. Most therapy groups focus on abstinence from alcohol as the treatment goal, although there might be some exceptions.

Why a Group?
Group therapy, in contrast to individual therapy, offers the opportunity to share experiences with and to learn from others. If you think you would like this, as opposed to meeting with a therapist on your own, check out a group. I can't recommend individual therapy over group therapy or vice versa, as I think it depends on your own personal preference. In contrast to self-help groups, group therapy will put greater emphasis on personal problems you have and how these may be playing a role in your drinking. Helping you work out particular concerns, learn healthier ways to cope, and improve difficult relationships can all be goals of group therapy.

Choose the Right Group

When considering group treatment, make sure that the focus of the group is to help people who have a problem with alcohol or drug abuse. A more general psychotherapy group will not focus on abstinence and learning how to accomplish this. If your goal is learning how to moderate your drinking, inform the group leader of this beforehand, because a group with the goal of abstinence will not be suitable for you. You should also think about whether you prefer to be in a group with both sexes or one with only members of your own sex. Again, ask about this if it's important to you. Many outpatient substance use treatment programs offer group therapy, and you can inquire about the availability of groups. Some private therapists also lead groups that might be appropriate for you.

PARTIAL HOSPITALIZATION AND INTENSIVE OUTPATIENT PROGRAMS

Partial hospitalization and intensive outpatient programs (IOPs) provide group treatment and support for people with an alcohol problem. These programs also offer individual therapy as well as educational and support meetings for family members. Most partial hospitalization and IOPs meet five or six days each week, from morning to mid- or late afternoon. Partial hospitalization programs generally meet for six hours each day, whereas IOPs meet for three hours each day. Partial hospitalization programs are more intensive, as they meet for a longer period of time, and they also have providers who can assess the need for medication. People can enter a partial hospitalization program first, when they believe they need more structure, and then later step down to an IOP; others may enter directly into an IOP. While the length of treatment is individualized, the programs generally last two to four weeks, or possibly a little longer.

All these programs offer a variety of psychoeducational and therapeutic groups, films, and discussions about aspects of substance abuse. Typical topics for group discussion include the following:

- the definition of an alcohol problem

- aspects of denial

- an alcohol problem as a family illness

- stress management

- dealing with urges

- leisure education and recreation

- coping with anger

- assertiveness training

- relapse warning signs and triggers

- relapse prevention

- introduction to self-help groups

- coping with painful feelings

Some specialized groups may also be offered, such as men's or women's groups, trauma groups, or groups for people who also have other psychiatric issues.

The goals of the program are to educate you about the nature of alcohol problems and to teach you the skills and coping mechanisms you need to achieve abstinence. You will learn about specific issues that may play a role in your inability to maintain abstinence and how to overcome your particular barriers to recovery.

Why Partial Hospitalization or an IOP?

These programs are indicated for you if you've tried less intensive forms of treatment, such as self-help meetings or weekly individual or group therapy, and haven't been able to achieve abstinence. These programs give you a lot of structure and can help you develop a new lifestyle that doesn't include drinking. This type of treatment builds a foundation so that you can achieve and maintain abstinence.

To find such a treatment program, your health insurance company will be able to provide you with information. You can also search online with the terms *alcoholism, alcohol treatment,* or *intensive outpatient treatment* to find a program in your area. If you have been seeing an individual therapist and are continuing to struggle with maintaining abstinence, that person could also recommend a partial hospitalization or IOP program. However, you need to make sure that your health insurance will pay for the recommended program.

EVENING TREATMENT PROGRAMS

Evening treatment programs, created to accommodate work schedules, are similar to IOPs in that they offer a structured group therapy program to enable you to achieve abstinence. Generally, an evening treatment program meets three or four times a week over several weeks, although the duration varies with the amount of treatment you need to resolve your problem. As with IOPs, evening treatment programs provide a variety of different groups and psychoeducational activities.

Why Evening Treatment?

If you work during the day, an evening treatment program will be more convenient for you than a daytime program. Evening treatment programs are more appropriate if you have already managed to maintain some periods of abstinence with an occasional relapse. While there are exceptions, evening treatment offers less structure than an IOP. These programs may meet less frequently during the week and for a shorter period of time. In general, if an IOP is a basic-training program, then evening treatment is a fine-tuning program.

Evening treatment will focus closely on your relapse triggers, and relapse prevention is typically a major focus of treatment. You can find out about such a program by calling your health insurance company or by searching online for *evening treatment program.* When inquiring, find out specifics about the program to determine whether it's appropriate for you.

RESIDENTIAL PROGRAMS

A residential program is any treatment program where you temporarily live on-site. These include inpatient detoxification programs, short-term rehabilitation (rehab) programs, halfway houses, and sober houses. Health insurance will pay for inpatient detoxification and short-term rehabilitation programs but not for halfway or sober houses.

As I discussed in chapter 6, some people will need to enter an inpatient detoxification program to be safely detoxified from alcohol. Quite often, after detoxification, a person may then enter a rehabilitation program for continued care. If you don't need detoxification but still need residential care because you haven't been able to achieve any significant periods of abstinence while living at home and having outpatient treatment, you often can enter such a program if you can demonstrate that you're not currently using alcohol or other drugs. Sometimes, though, to ensure that you are safe and do not require detoxification, a program will recommend that you get admitted to an observation bed, where you will be medically monitored for a short time until cleared to step down to a rehabilitation program.

If you don't have health insurance, there are some residential treatment programs. Another option is to pay for the services with your own money. You can get information on specific programs in your area through your state department of health, which will probably have an alcohol or substance use disorder division that maintains a list of all facilities. Other alcohol and drug use disorder treatment programs will also have this information available.

Another great resource for finding a residential program, or any type of alcohol treatment program, is http://findtreatment.samhsa .gov, a website sponsored by the federal Substance Abuse and Mental Health Services Administration. This site lists all drug and alcohol facilities in the United States, and you can find an appropriate program by clicking on the substance abuse treatment facility locator.

Be an Informed Consumer

Before I discuss inpatient detoxification and short-term rehab programs, which can be of enormous assistance to you when you require medical detoxification or cannot resolve your drinking problem on an outpatient basis, you must be aware that badly run programs do exist. While many, if not most, are well designed and well run, there are some that look good on the surface but that offer deficient treatment. In some cases these deficiencies can border on being unethical, in my opinion.

The opioid epidemic has created additional detoxification and rehab programs because so many individuals have required professional inpatient treatment to address their addiction to heroin or prescription opioids. Where there is a growing demand for services, the market will grow to meet the need. As a result, the number of available programs has expanded, and these programs obviously need admissions to cover their expenses. Many of these programs are well intentioned and designed to treat their customers ethically in all services. However, some programs that originally opened to help individuals have, over time, shifted their focus to making money by ensuring that their beds stay occupied.

It is important for you to be an informed consumer so that you get the treatment you want. Let me share with you some things to be aware of when assessing an inpatient substance use disorder treatment program, which generally includes a detoxification and post-detoxification or rehab program. It is not my intention to dissuade you from entering such a program. Rather, it is my desire that you have a positive and worthwhile treatment experience.

Know What You Are Getting Into. To begin with, when considering an admission to such a program, do not be bashful. Feel free to ask any and all questions that you have—about the kind of treatment offered, the type of staff and the staff's credentials, accommodations, dietary needs or restrictions that you have, what a typical day is like, visiting hours and policies, opportunities to make phone calls, what exercise or outdoor activities are available, or anything else that is important to you. Some individuals may need to keep up with work, so you can also ask whether you can have access to a computer or telephone. While you need to focus on yourself when in such a program, some people may need to keep up with some outside work commitments, and accommodations can be made for that.

The cost of treatment should also be made clear up front so that you know what you will be responsible to pay for. Insurance policies are all different, and programs can check to see what if any deductible you have to meet or what copay or other charges may fall to you. There can be some add-on services that may not be covered by your insurance, so ask about that as well.

Prior to calling a particular treatment program, you can check with your insurance company to see what programs are in-network as opposed to those that are out-of-network. In-network programs are those that your insurance company has a relationship with and that typically will cost you less than an out-of-network program.

There may be times when a program tells you something not entirely accurate to get you to enroll. If there are certain things quite important to you, such as having access to a computer for work, I would encourage you to get something in writing from the program that details its policies or that guarantees your access to something. This way, there will be no misunderstanding when you are in the program, which will only distract you from your purpose for being there. The program should not hesitate in giving you anything in writing. If it refuses, I would consider finding someplace else.

How Long Are You Willing to Be in Treatment? Another important consideration for many people is the length of time they will remain in inpatient treatment. The time it takes to be detoxified from alcohol is generally one week or less. After detoxification, many people choose to spend some time in a rehab. Time in rehab can allow your body to heal; it gives you additional time away from your living environment, where you may be tempted to drink again; and you learn skills you need to remain abstinent from alcohol.

The length of your stay should be based on the severity of your alcohol problem and other possible life challenges, such as your psychological status and the quality of your social support at home. The length of stay should also take into account your willingness and desire to be in treatment. Unfortunately, in the interest of making money, some programs will recommend a longer stay for everyone, without conducting a good assessment or taking your wishes into account.

Convey Your Intentions. At the time of admission to a program, you may not be sure how long you wish to remain in treatment after detoxification, so you may be willing to take a "wait and see" approach. Others, though, may have an idea of how long they can stay in treatment on account of other things they have going on in their lives. If you have a time limit, you should communicate that information at the outset of treatment. You can always change your mind once in treatment, especially if you decide to stay longer, but letting the staff know how long you are willing to stay prior to admission is a good idea.

I suggest that you convey your intentions prior to admission and get something in writing. In programs that are focused on filling beds, once you are in treatment, the staff may pressure you to stay in treatment for as long as possible, *or for as long as your health insurance is willing to pay for you to be in treatment.* While a longer stay may be appropriate for some people, this is not true for everyone. People who do not wish to stay in treatment too long and who feel forced to be there will benefit less from being in treatment. Making your expectations clear at the outset will help you avoid a situation where you feel pressured to remain in treatment when you don't want to be.

Speak with Your Loved One(s). I would also advise you to share with your loved ones your plans for how long you wish to remain in treatment. Making your plans known will help you avoid any tension when your discharge is approaching. You do not want to be in a situation where you plan to be in treatment for two weeks and your loved ones think you will be in treatment for a month or longer. There may be cases when you cannot agree, which is another matter that may need to be worked out over time when you are in treatment.

Assuming that you are in agreement, telling your loved ones your plan may prevent any conflict if your treatment provider contacts a loved one (provided that you have consented to such communication) and recommends that you stay in treatment for a longer period of time than you originally agreed to. For a program focused on filling beds, and contrary to your wishes, staff may try to convince your loved one that you need stay in treatment longer. Staff might claim that you are minimizing or denying your problem and that a longer stay is necessary.

In such a situation, your loved one may be tempted to agree with your provider. Your loved one may even refuse to allow you to return home until your treatment provider states that it is fine for you to be discharged. This can cause enormous tension between you and your loved ones. Having communicated clear expectations will help you avoid a disagreement about the length of treatment when discharge is approaching. You may want to warn your loved ones prior to entering treatment that they may get a call from the rehab center encouraging them to convince you to stay in treatment longer. Knowing this could occur can prepare them to handle such a call with more composure and rational thinking.

Outpatient Programs That Are More Like Inpatient Programs. A newer development in the field, often known as the Florida Model, is having clients live on-site at the program while attending an outpatient program, such as a partial hospitalization or an IOP. These programs allow people to attend the outpatient program who live far away or who do not have a stable place to live. The Florida Model is also a way to extend treatment on a quasi-inpatient basis, because, quite commonly, individuals attending the outpatient program live on the grounds and must submit to rules and structure that mimic an inpatient program.

Such a program will charge a patient's insurance company for the cost of the partial hospitalization program and will allow the patient to live there at no cost. Once the person steps down to the IOP, which again will be billed to the person's insurance company, that individual will then be expected to pay a nominal fee for living at the program. This is done because the insurance reimbursement for the partial hospitalization program is more than that for the IOP.

For some individuals, this provides a great opportunity to remain in a structured treatment program without having to deal with the stresses of returning to their home environment. While in treatment, they can continue to work on building the skills they need to remain free from alcohol. For others, however, this may feel too confining, as they prefer to return to home sooner and attend a partial hospitalization or IOP closer to where they live. There is no right or wrong choice for all; people are different, and each person should do what he or she thinks is best.

Treatment Success and Outcome. Finally, you can also ask a program about its treatment success. In truth, though, such statistics are difficult to ascertain. Programs find it hard to conduct good follow-up with former patients. When assessing treatment success, the big question is how long after treatment has patient success been measured. One-month or three-month post-treatment success is much different from measuring rates of abstinence at six months or a year after treatment. If a program's statistics sound too good to be true, they likely are, and you should be suspicious. On the other hand, an ethical program will likely tell you that this is hard data to collect, and the program may give you some ideas about what it has found when trying to assess this.

Satisfaction surveys, which ask patients how satisfied they were with the care they received, are another measure that some providers may share with you. You can also look at reviews online to get a sense of what people are saying about the program. You can even ask the program what things it has done to improve the care it provides. Continuous performance improvement should be a practice at any program, and a program should be able to tell you what it has done to enhance its services.

Do Not Be Intimidated. My intention in laying out concerns about residential programs is not to discourage you from entering such a program when you want to or feel you need to. I am a big believer in treatment, which has helped millions of people. In fact, I have clinically overseen many treatment programs in my career, and I and the people I worked with all strove hard to offer the best possible care. Rather, my aim is to ensure that you choose an ethical and well-run program that has your interests at the forefront of anything it does. My aim is also to help you get the treatment that you want, that meets your needs, and most important, that enables you to achieve your goals. Let me now describe what rehab is and why you might consider it.

Rehabilitation Programs

A rehabilitation program, rehab for short, provides intensive education and structure in a residential setting. In such settings, groups, films, discussions, and AA or other self-help meetings are offered to teach you the skills you need to attain and maintain abstinence. One-to-one counseling is also available that gives you the opportunity to look closely at yourself and your alcohol problem. The time you spend in a residential program can vary from several weeks to a couple of months, or until an appropriate discharge plan has been developed. While some rehabs are coed, others may be only for men or only for women.

Why a Rehab Facility? Rehabilitation programs can be helpful if you have been unable to benefit from other less-structured forms of treatment and it is clear that you need a lot of education and skill building to attain abstinence. A rehab will provide you with a time out from your usual way of life and your usual friends, and it will give you the opportunity to work intensely on yourself so that you can develop the skills you need to remain abstinent. A rehab will also ensure that you do not drink while you reside in a structured, contained environment. This kind of program is appropriate if you have limited social support (few or no sober people in your life) to foster abstinence. If you have been unable to achieve abstinence using other resources, you should consider such a program.

Halfway Houses

A halfway house is a residential treatment program that provides longer-term support. Many people enter a halfway house after first being in a rehab. The term *halfway* implies that the program is halfway between the community and the treatment world. Often, while living at a halfway house, you can work at a job nearby, although some programs may restrict outside work. Halfway houses may be partially supported by state funds, which defray the cost of treatment until residents can afford to pay rent to live there, just as anyone pays rent or a mortgage to live in an apartment or home. Others have no other funding, and residents are expected to pay to live there as soon as they move in.

Halfway houses differ in their degree of structure. Some houses restrict privileges for several weeks after a person is admitted. For example, new residents may not be able to leave the grounds without being accompanied by a staff member or a longer-term resident of the program, and obtaining an outside job may not be allowed or only allowed after a period of time. Other halfway houses immediately or soon allow and encourage residents to resume employment. How much free time is allowed also varies, as does the amount of treatment offered. Some houses have frequent in-house meetings, require residents to attend AA or other self-help meetings in the community, and have residents take saliva and urine tests to monitor alcohol or drug use. Others offer and require less formal treatment.

How long you live in a halfway house also varies based on your need for continued treatment and on the structure of the program. In general, a stay lasts for several months or even a year. When contacting a halfway house for possible admission, ask about the rules and requirements of the program to ensure that you are entering the type of program you want. Be an informed consumer.

As with rehabs, some halfway houses are coed, but others may be just for men or just for women. There are also some specialized halfway houses, although they are not as numerous. For example, some are only for adolescents, others are primarily for gay or transgender individuals, and others are designed for women who want to live there with their children.

Why a Halfway House? A halfway house is useful if you have a serious alcohol problem and require intensive and long-term treatment to stay sober. These programs offer a living environment that is free of alcohol, and this can be particularly helpful if you don't have a living arrangement that supports your abstinent lifestyle. Because all residents in a halfway house are attempting to achieve abstinence, you can get considerable peer support. The feeling that *we are all in this together, trying to get our lives together by not drinking* can be quite powerful, and it helps to counter the notion that you are struggling all alone against the world.

You should consider this type of program if you repeatedly have been unable to achieve abstinence in the community and if people in your home drink immoderately. After you leave a short-term rehab, a halfway house may help you build a foundation for long-term abstinence.

Sober Houses

A sober house is similar to a halfway house in that a group of individuals who are all trying to achieve abstinence live together in a home and provide support to one another. However, sober houses offer less structure and treatment than halfway houses.

Sober houses are often used as a step-down after an individual completes a halfway house program. Individuals also can enter them directly from the community or from an inpatient detoxification or rehabilitation program. Some sober houses offer little, if any, formalized treatment or structure, whereas others expect you to attend house meetings like halfway houses often do. Some may require attendance at outside self-help meetings, as well as submitting to random saliva or urine tests to monitor alcohol or drug use, so be sure to inquire about this. Sober houses are supported by the residents who pay rent to live there.

Why a Sober House? Like halfway houses, a sober house can provide a support system to help you get back on your feet and achieve long-term abstinence. You should consider such a program if you have been unable to maintain abstinence on your own, your home situation does not support a nondrinking lifestyle, and you feel that you could benefit from living with others who are also trying not to drink.

SUMMARY

In this chapter, I reviewed the range of professional treatment services available should you find you need additional support to address your drinking problem. The treatment options vary in their intensity and the support they offer—from residential treatment programs (the most intensive), to partial hospitalization and IOPs, to once-a-week outpatient individual, group, or marital and family therapy.

The type of treatment that makes the most sense for you depends on the severity of your drinking problem and on your living situation. If you find that once-a-week outpatient therapy is not working for you because your drinking continues to be problematic, that is a sign you should consider a partial hospitalization program or an IOP, which offers more structure and support. If you then find that option is not helping either, you should consider rehab and perhaps further residential treatment after rehab. The key is never to give up.

CHAPTER 18

Medications

The brain is the most complex object of human inquiry.
James H. Billington, DPhil, Librarian of Congress,
and Steven E. Hyman, MD, Director, National Institute
of Mental Health

During the last 30 years or so, there has been an explosion in our knowledge of the brain. Technologies have been developed that help us better understand how this complex organ works, including some ideas about how alcohol interacts with the brain, what it is about alcohol that makes people want to drink it, and why alcohol can be hard to quit. As a result, some new medications have been produced specifically for the treatment of an alcohol problem.

There are currently three types of medication approved by the US Food and Drug Administration (FDA) and available to people with an alcohol problem who want to stop drinking:

• Antabuse (disulfiram)

• ReVia (naltrexone)

• Campral (acamprosate)

Disulfiram has been around a long time, but naltrexone and acamprosate are much newer. These medications work in quite different ways, and all three must be prescribed by a physician or an advanced practice nurse who is able to prescribe medication.

As alcohol problems are complex and these medications work in such different ways, there has been some research into whether taking two of these drugs together can have an even greater benefit.

While not many studies have looked into this, the results of the ones that have did not demonstrate an additional benefit from taking two of these medications together.

The recommendation for how long to take these medications is at least three months, the period of time when the chance of a relapse is highest. However, these medications often can be taken for one year or even longer. You and your doctor can decide what might be best for you.

There are also several medications that are being used off-label to help people with a drinking problem. *Off-label* means that an FDA-approved drug is being prescribed for an unapproved use, such as using the medication for a different condition, at a different dosage, or sometimes with a population different from the one it was approved for. These medications have likely shown benefit in some small studies but are not yet approved by the FDA for these other indications.

Before I discuss each of these medications, the most important thing you need to know is that they are all *tools* to help you stop drinking. None is a *total treatment program.* If you are still struggling to stay sober, don't think that simply taking a medication will turn everything around for you. In American society there is a belief that most any problem can be solved with a pill. You have a cold? Take a drug. You want to lose weight? Take a drug. Feeling stressed? Here's a drug. And the list goes on and on. Although the medications mentioned here can be extremely helpful, it takes more than medication alone to overcome an alcohol problem. As you've learned, recovery is a lifestyle change, and medication cannot, nor is designed to, do that.

DISULFIRAM (ANTABUSE)

Disulfiram is a drug that discourages you from drinking. If you take disulfiram and drink, you'll become quite ill. Symptoms include flushing of the skin, a throbbing headache, nausea or even vomiting, sweating, anxiety, chest pain, palpitations, and hyperventilation and respiratory distress. An extreme reaction can bring on shock and cardiac arrhythmia.

How It Works

When a person consumes alcohol, the liver breaks it down into *acetaldehyde* with an enzyme called *alcohol dehydrogenase*. Acetaldehyde is then converted into acetic acid by *acetaldehyde dehydrogenase*, but disulfiram blocks the breakdown of acetaldehyde in the bloodstream. Acetaldehyde is very toxic and causes the alcohol-disulfiram reaction I just described.

If you take disulfiram, the fear of experiencing a painful reaction to alcohol stops you from drinking. If you take disulfiram every day, you don't seriously consider drinking because you know, beyond a doubt, that if you drink, you will get wretchedly sick.

Of course, the protection against drinking that disulfiram provides works only if you take it. If you aren't motivated to stop drinking, you'll find a way not to. Maybe you'll "forget" to take it. And, inevitably, at some point in the not-too-distant future, you'll start to drink again. Even if you don't admit it to yourself, you probably stopped taking it because you made the decision to drink again.

You must be highly motivated to stop drinking if you take disulfiram because you know that mixing the two will make you sick. You should be aware that a reaction to disulfiram can occur up to 14 days after the last dose is taken.

Things to Know

Disulfiram should be initiated after a person has completed alcohol withdrawal. Because disulfiram reacts highly to alcohol, you need to be careful to avoid all types of alcohol. For example, you should not eat pastry or candy that contains alcohol. In fact, you shouldn't do this anyway because, regardless of where alcohol comes from, you need to avoid it—period. You don't want to eat or drink any alcohol, since taking even a tiny amount can escalate to your ingesting more and more, as reviewed in chapters 10 and 13. You also need to avoid products like mouthwash, cough syrups, or other medications that contain alcohol. There is also a small risk of having a disulfiram reaction to aftershave lotions and perfumes that contain alcohol, so you need to read labels carefully. Your doctor can review with you the things you need to avoid.

On the other hand, if you eat food in which alcohol was used in the cooking process, the alcohol has usually evaporated, so this should not be a problem. Pastries with vanilla extract, for example, should not be problem. If excessive amounts of alcohol have been used, however, like wine in some sauces, some alcohol can remain, which could cause a reaction. In general, it is better to be more cautious rather than less.

As with all medications, there can be some side effects to disulfiram, most of which are generally mild. In addition, not everyone can take disulfiram for medical reasons. Only your physician can decide whether disulfiram is suitable for you. If you are interested in trying disulfiram, speak with your physician, who can answer your specific questions. If you are highly motivated to stop drinking, you can consider this medication, along with all of the other things you can do to help yourself.

NALTREXONE (REVIA)

Naltrexone is a much newer agent than disulfiram and works in a significantly different way. Rather than making you sick if you drink alcohol, it can help take away a craving for alcohol. If you do drink, you won't experience the same feelings of intoxication that you used to, so it may keep you from experiencing a relapse, as you won't want to drink more and more.

How It Works

Endorphins are naturally occurring opioids that we all have in our bodies. Opioids are painkillers, and these natural opioids cause euphoria, sedation, and a sense of well-being when they attach to certain areas in the brain called receptor sites.

When you drink, endorphins are released and attach to the receptor sites in your brain that cause the pleasurable feelings you get by drinking. One way to help a person who struggles with an alcohol problem is to prevent endorphins from attaching to those receptor sites. If this is done, alcohol will no longer have the same effect, so the person won't want to drink as much. Naltrexone does just this. If you drink while taking naltrexone, you won't feel the usual euphoria, pleasure, and well-being. As you no longer get the same kick from drinking, you won't want to drink, or at least you won't want to drink as much.

Research has found that people who took naltrexone reported drinking less than people who did not take it, and when they drank, they suffered a relapse less often. Interestingly enough, people who took naltrexone also reported significantly less craving for alcohol than people who were not taking it. Exactly how naltrexone decreases craving is not entirely clear, but it does appear to have this effect. So if you struggle with intense cravings and urges to drink, I strongly recommend that you give naltrexone a try. Naltrexone is prescribed to help people achieve abstinence, but because naltrexone has been shown to decrease days of heavy drinking, it is also prescribed to people who are trying to reduce their drinking.

There is also an injectable form of naltrexone called Vivitrol that works in the same way but lasts for an entire month. A doctor can give you a shot. The advantage of taking naltrexone this way is that you don't have to remember to take it every day but only have to remember to see your doctor monthly. This is a good alternative for you if you don't like to take a daily pill or don't think you'll remember to take it every day.

Things to Know

As with all medications, naltrexone can have some side effects, but these are generally mild. There are also some individuals who should not take naltrexone because of a medical condition. In particular, if you have significant liver disease or elevated liver enzymes, you can't take naltrexone. If you are interested in trying this medication, make an appointment with your physician to see if it's right for you.

You should also know that because naltrexone blocks all opioids from attaching to those receptor sites, it will prevent opioid drugs from acting in the body. This means that if you take an opioid pain-killer for an injury or other reason, it won't work. You will have to use another drug or other method to control pain instead. Your doctor can discuss this with you and suggest other pain medications you can take.

Naltrexone has been shown to be effective among people who have been able to abstain from alcohol in an outpatient setting prior to initiating naltrexone treatment. Contrarily, naltrexone has not been shown to be effective in patients who were drinking at the time they started taking the drug.

ACAMPROSATE (CAMPRAL)

Acamprosate is another medication used to treat people with alcohol problems. Like naltrexone, acamprosate helps reduce the cravings you can experience when you first stop drinking. As a result, acamprosate is best prescribed right after you stop using alcohol, and it seems to work best for individuals who are abstinent when prescribed it. So, if you experience strong cravings to use, especially right after you stop drinking, you should consider acamprosate.

How It Works

It is not entirely clear how acamprosate works, but it has something to do with restoring the imbalance of chemicals (*neurotransmitters*) in your brain that can be caused by heavy drinking. A number of studies conducted in Europe and the United States have shown that rates of abstinence were greater among people who took acamprosate than among people who took a placebo. In addition, the total number of days of not drinking was higher among the people who took acamprosate.

Things to Know

As with disulfiram and naltrexone, acamprosate needs to be prescribed by a physician, and there are some people who can't take this medication for medical reasons. For example, some individuals are hypersensitive to the drug and experience an allergic reaction to it. Those with severe renal impairment cannot take it either. Your physician can determine whether this drug is indicated for you.

OFF-LABEL MEDICATIONS

Topiramate

Topiramate is a medication that is used to prevent seizures and migraine headaches but that has also been found to help people with their drinking. Studies have found that it increased the proportion of people who were able to achieve abstinence or days of non-heavy drinking. Unlike some other medications, topiramate was found to work even for people who were still drinking when they first started taking it. The precise mechanism of its action is not clear, but it helps to restore the balance of neurotransmission in the brain. It is taken orally, and the dose is gradually increased to minimize any side effects.

Gabapentin

Gabapentin is a medication that is used to treat epileptic seizures and neuropathic pain. Some studies have shown that gabapentin improved rates of abstinence and decreased days of heavy drinking. Gabapentin was also found to enhance mood, improve sleep, and decrease craving. A higher dose seemed to be more effective than a lower dose, and there were no adverse effects from a higher dose.

Exactly how gabapentin improved rates of abstinence and decreased days of heavy drinking is not clear. However, it is believed to work by decreasing stress-induced activation of some neurotransmitter systems in the brain associated with alcohol dependence. It is taken orally and, like all the medications described in this chapter, needs to be prescribed by a physician or other health care professional authorized to prescribe medication.

Varenicline

Varenicline is a medication that is used to help people stop smoking, and there is some evidence that it may help people decrease alcohol intake as well. Several studies of varenicline in heavy-drinking smokers in treatment for their smoking found that the medication decreased their alcohol consumption, although it did not improve rates of abstinence. There was also some evidence that it may help decrease cravings for alcohol. The medication is believed to work on certain receptor sites in the brain involved in the rewarding effects of alcohol. Although most of the studies had patients who drank and smoked, this medication may be help individuals who drink excessively but don't smoke.

PSYCHIATRIC MEDICATIONS

In chapter 17, I mentioned that some people who stop drinking continue to feel bad, and I suggested individual or group psychotherapy. There are times, though, when therapy alone may not be enough. Psychiatric medication can be prescribed to treat symptoms that are unrelated to a person's alcohol problem.

It is quite common for problem drinkers to have other psychiatric problems. In fact, a study conducted by the National Institute of Mental Health found that among people who have ever experienced an alcohol problem, a little over one-third had experienced a psychiatric disorder at some point in their lives. Common psychiatric problems were depression, anxiety, and bipolar disorder, which is a mood disorder characterized by feelings of extreme highs and lows. In fact, the chance of someone with an alcohol problem having a psychiatric disorder is about double that of people who have never had an alcohol problem.

Fortunately, many medications target neurochemical processes in our brains that relate to psychiatric complaints. A psychiatrist or other trained health care professional can determine whether a particular medication should be taken for a psychological difficulty, although other mental health professionals such as psychologists and social workers often have a pretty good sense of when medication may be needed. Such individuals make referrals to prescribers who will determine whether medication makes sense and what type of medication should be prescribed.

Who Doesn't Need Medication

Many people who stop drinking may suffer from some emotional distress but don't need and should not be prescribed medication. Their solution involves learning new ways to cope that don't include alcohol. For example, at the time you decide to do something about your drinking problem, you may feel miserable, awful, and down. You may also be anxious about the current problems in your life, many of which may have been caused by your drinking. This is further compounded by the fact that you must now deal with these problems without alcohol, your usual way of coping.

So, initially, you may feel troubled and overwhelmed when you first stop drinking. Your solution, though, is learning how to manage your problems without drinking, either on your own or with the support of therapy. As you do this, you'll find that, pretty quickly, you start to feel better without turning to medication. If you have had past periods of not drinking, and life was good and you felt good, that is a probable sign that you do not need medication.

Who Needs Medication

For some people, medication is an essential treatment intervention if they are ever going to feel better. For example, without medication, people with bipolar disorder will continue to experience intense mood swings that will make their lives unmanageable. Without stabilizing their moods, it can be difficult or impossible for them to abstain from alcohol. Such people *need* medication as a component of their recovery program.

While bipolar disorder is a serious psychiatric condition, others experience more subtle difficulties that also require medication. You may have resolved your drinking problem and made the necessary changes to support your new life, yet you may continue to feel mildly or severely depressed. I have seen many people who report feelings of depression and can't pinpoint why they continue to feel so miserable. Often they report that things in their lives are good and that, despite having no reason to feel bad, they still do. Medication can help to resolve those feelings so that they can enjoy life again.

To assess whether a medication evaluation makes sense for people who continue to feel "off," I will ask them if they have been abstinent in the past for a good period of time, such as 6 to 12 months. If they have and they continued to feel bad, this suggests that an evaluation for medication is indicated. So for you, if you are no longer drinking and still feel bad, and have previously not felt right despite not drinking, I would encourage you to consider making an appointment for a medication evaluation.

Other people may experience considerable difficulty getting a handle on their drinking problem due, in part, to their depression. Medication can play an important role in enabling these people to finally resolve their drinking problem. So if you are working hard to make the lifestyle changes that go along with not drinking, but you continue to feel bad or maybe even lapse after feeling awful, consider medication.

Most important, don't think that nothing can be done, that it's your fault you continue to feel bad, or that you are doing something wrong. Your effort may have nothing to do with it, and you should make an appointment to see a psychiatrist, who can determine whether some type of medication makes sense for you.

For some of you, this may be a big step. It may be hard to admit you need this help, or you may view it as a crutch. But try not to see it that way. Instead, accept that certain people need medication to feel better. It's just that simple. For many psychiatric disorders, medication is the treatment of choice, just as insulin is for the treatment of diabetes or as antibiotics are for the treatment of an infection. A psychiatrist who is knowledgeable about alcohol problems can determine whether medication might benefit you.

You should also know that sleep difficulties can sometimes occur after a person stops drinking. Fortunately, they often go away in a fairly short period of time and do not cause the person too much distress. However, there are others who continue to struggle with falling asleep, staying asleep, or waking up too early in the morning. If sleep difficulties continue to affect you, there are medications that can help. However, be sure to tell your prescriber about your alcohol problem because there are certain sleep medications you should not take.

When to Start Medication

Professionals in psychotherapy used to think that people with a drinking problem should not be prescribed psychiatric medication for at least six months to a year after resolving their drinking problem. This practice stemmed from the belief that a person could not be properly diagnosed with an emotional disorder until alcohol had been out of their system for a long period of time. This is no longer the belief, however, and doctors do prescribe medication even shortly after a person has stopped drinking. If you need medication, yet delay starting it, you will have a lower chance of achieving abstinence. Or even if you are able to stop drinking, you will continue to feel bad.

On the other hand, it is impossible to know if you need medication if your drinking remains out of control. Alcohol is a powerful drug and can affect how you feel. For example, if you feel depressed, your drinking may be responsible for these feelings, or at least it contributes to them. So while medication can be started early on, a short period of abstinence is needed to make a proper diagnosis and decision about whether medication should be prescribed. Even if you feel bad and think that drinking helps you cope, you owe it to yourself to take a break from drinking so that you can be properly evaluated.

Things to Know

If you see a psychiatrist for a medication evaluation, be sure to tell the person that you have struggled with alcohol consumption because certain medications should not be prescribed to you (some sleeping aids, as I mentioned). Some medications have the potential to be misused, particularly by people who have a history of excessive alcohol or drug use. Your psychiatrist will also review with you the potential problems of drinking while taking a prescribed medication.

If you are prescribed medication for a psychiatric problem, this doesn't mean that your alcohol problem is no longer important or doesn't still need your focus and attention. Your psychiatric problem, while it may have played a role in the development of your alcohol problem and may continue to have an influence on it, is not entirely responsible for your alcohol problem. Both problems exist, and you must address them both. Even when your psychiatric problem is properly treated and you're feeling better, your alcohol problem doesn't go away. You still have a predilection to drink too much, and you need to focus on this.

SUMMARY

If you continue to struggle with being unable to resolve your drinking problem, or if you continue to feel bad despite no longer drinking, there are a number of medications that could help you. The brain is a very complicated organ, and there is still much we do not understand about its function. However, we have learned a lot, and research has shown that some medications can help a person achieve sobriety. There are medications designed to help you with your alcohol problem, and other medications can treat psychiatric problems you may experience.

Do not feel bad if you require medication for additional support. These medications have been developed to help you and others who continue to struggle despite their best efforts. At the same time, never forget that medication is not a total treatment program. Medication can support you, but you must still do your part. It is the combination of your work and medication that will get you to where you want to be.

PART VI

Other Drug Use
in Recovery

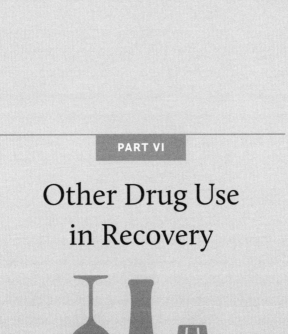

CHAPTER 19

Can You Smoke Marijuana?

Pay attention to your body. The point is everybody is different.
You have to figure out what works for you.
ANDREW WEIL

A question that often arises when I work with people who have struggled with alcohol is whether they can use a different substance such as marijuana. That is, if they are abstinent from alcohol or are drinking in a controlled way, it is possible for them to use marijuana? I am not talking about excessive marijuana use but about using it in a way that does not harm them or others or that interferes with their ability to lead a successful and productive life. Individuals who wonder about this are typically those who have used marijuana along with alcohol, as opposed to people who never used marijuana.

I am not talking about the use of cannabidiol, or CBD, but rather delta-9-tetrahydrocannabinol, or THC. THC is the psychoactive ingredient in marijuana that causes euphoria or a "high" feeling. CBD, on the other hand, is not psychoactive but does have a calming or anxiety-reducing effect. It can help people fall and stay asleep and may also be useful in reducing seizures in certain types of epilepsy.

Wanting to alter one's consciousness is likely a universal human desire. Throughout history, people have done things to change their ordinary way of being in the world. It is reported that an alcoholic drink existed in China around 7000 BC. In India, there is evidence of production of an alcoholic beverage between 3000 and 2000 BC, and around 2700 BC the Babylonians worshipped a wine goddess. It is believed that, about 2,500 years ago, marijuana was used for its psychogenic effects in central Asia. Opium production and use has been dated to around 3400 BC in southwestern Asia, and the poppy plant, from which opium is derived, was often referred to as the "joy plant."

While using alcohol and drugs is one easy way to alter consciousness, other ways that may take more initiative and work include meditation, sleep deprivation, bungee jumping, going on a scary ride, or experiencing other peak experiences like rock climbing or parachuting. Other more subtle ways include immersing oneself in an engaging novel, watching an entertaining movie, running, bicycle riding, or taking a walk in the woods or along the beach. Even young children enjoy altering their consciousness when they spin around and around to make themselves dizzy. Some children love to be thrown up in the air or turned upside down to experience a different sensation.

That many people still wish to alter their ordinary state of being after they stop using alcohol for this purpose does not surprise me. Ideally, people should learn how to change their ordinary way of being in the world through healthy activities, without resorting to substance use. Using a substance, though, can be appealing because it enables people to change their perception quickly and with little effort, which is why the question of marijuana use often arises. Without condoning alcohol or marijuana use, I find that some people can occasionally use a substance to change their mental state without it having a negative impact on their lives, whereas others cannot.

Whether former drinkers can safely use marijuana to get high has become a more frequently asked question with the availability of medical marijuana and the legalization of marijuana for recreational use in some states. The issue is whether using marijuana can jeopardize a recovery from alcohol misuse. Does using marijuana lead people back to excessive alcohol use, or will people begin to misuse marijuana over time?

To answer these questions is challenging for many reasons. First, as I have maintained throughout this book, alcohol and other substance use disorders are multifaceted. They vary along a continuum of severity and are determined by many factors. Everyone is different, and there is no one size that fits all. For some, using marijuana could lead them back to problematic drinking, whereas for others it may not. It is also possible that using marijuana could become problematic in and of itself. Certainly, people can become dependent on marijuana, which can affect the quality of their life.

Research in this area is not well established. While some studies have looked at using other drugs while in recovery, there is still a lot we do not know, which makes it hard to give definitive recommendations. Critically, there have been no studies of treatment interventions for people who struggle with alcohol and who want to smoke marijuana to help them keep their alcohol and marijuana use in control. Despite this, I can share what I have seen in my clinical work, review some research on this issue, and offer some tentative recommendations.

WHAT I HAVE OBSERVED

Nonproblematic Drug Use

During my career as a therapist, I have worked with people who had a range of substance use problems beyond alcohol, including problems with heroin, prescription opioids, and cocaine or other stimulant drugs. Many of these people also smoked marijuana. As I mentioned in the introduction of this book, I was originally trained to believe that complete abstinence was the only way to recover from an alcohol problem, a belief that extended to drugs as well. And for people who used multiple drugs, abstinence from all drugs was essential if they were going to get better. The thinking was that "a drug is a drug is a drug," and abstinence was recommended for any substance a person used or ever would consider using. There was no such thing as any drug or alcohol use in recovery.

Much to my surprise, I have seen people who resolved their primary substance use problem but continued to use another substance safely. Here are some examples:

- Chris, a 28-year-old single man, readily admitted that he used to have a cocaine problem. He stopped using cocaine but occasionally drank and smoked marijuana without it affecting him negatively.

- Jennifer, a 32-year-old single woman who worked successfully as a manager of a retail store, had resolved her problem with opiates several years ago. Currently, she would occasionally drink, which consisted of having a couple of glasses of wine.

- Rob, a married 34-year-old man, used to go to bars, where he would drink way too much and use cocaine excessively only when he got very intoxicated. He was able to resolve both his alcohol and cocaine problem by learning to moderate his drinking. He had always smoked some marijuana, never saw it as a problem, and continued to smoke marijuana occasionally as well.

- Mark, a 37-year-old married man with two children, resolved his problem with alcohol by achieving abstinence, but he would still occasionally smoke marijuana when he got together with some friends who smoked it.

- Sue, a 42-year-old married woman who had gotten addicted to heroin in her youth, now occasionally drank small amounts of alcohol without any difficulties. She did not smoke marijuana, though, because she did not like the way it made her feel.

These people told me that smoking marijuana or drinking alcohol was simply not a big deal. It was something they did occasionally, but it just never had grabbed them the way their drug of choice did. They did not struggle to control their current alcohol or marijuana use, and it did not lead them back to their prior problematic drug or alcohol use. These people made me realize that there were some for whom abstinence from all drugs did not appear to be necessary for their recovery.

Problematic Drug Use

On the other hand, I have also worked with people who continued to use or began to use other drugs when in recovery, and things did not go well. Here are some examples:

- Kathy, a 44-year-old single woman, had struggled with heroin off and on for much of her life. When she was able to attain abstinence from heroin, she would soon begin to drink alcohol and smoke marijuana occasionally, and within a fairly short period of time, she relapsed into heroin use. This had happened to her numerous times. She was finally able to see that she needed to abstain from all drugs and alcohol if she was ever going to resolve her heroin problem.

- Jim, a 34-year-old single man, who had a long-term heroin problem, was often able to put together long periods of abstinence from heroin, despite continuing to smoke marijuana, which he thought was OK to do. However, he had experienced many relapses into heroin, and over time he began to see that his marijuana use contributed to this. He then decided to stop smoking marijuana entirely.

- John, a 29-year-old married man with a young son, struggled with alcohol and smoked a lot of marijuana. He initially decided to stop both his alcohol and marijuana use. After one month of abstaining from alcohol and marijuana, he decided to smoke marijuana again, and over the course of the next month, he found himself drinking again. He was able to see that his marijuana use was a factor in his drinking. He decided that if he was going to resolve his drinking problem, he needed to abstain from marijuana as well.

- Justin, a 37-year-old single man, came to treatment because his girlfriend was fed up with his excessive substance use and no longer wanted to see him. He knew he had an alcohol problem but did not feel that his marijuana use was an issue, although he smoked a lot of it. He decided to stop drinking and made the decision to limit his use of marijuana. Despite this intention, he continued to smoke marijuana quite heavily. When his girlfriend continued to complain about his excessive marijuana use, he was able to see how it was affecting him and his relationship, and he realized that he also needed to stop smoking marijuana.

Unlike those who found they could occasionally take another substance without it affecting their recovery, these people discovered that any drug use was problematic for them. They found that occasional use of another substance undermined their recovery from their primary substance problem, or they learned that the secondary substance they continued to use became troublesome for them too. Frequently they discovered that using any substance led to an obsession with using substances again, whether the secondary substance, the primary substance, or both. They realized that abstinence from all substances was the only solution.

WHAT THE RESEARCH SHOWS

While the research is relatively sparse on the impact of continued marijuana use on substance use treatment outcome, it mirrors what I have seen in my practice. Some researchers have found no relationship between marijuana use and overall treatment outcome. In fact, one study showed that marijuana use enhanced treatment outcome for individuals seeking help for crack cocaine addiction. However, other studies found that ongoing marijuana use was associated with a poorer treatment outcome. Many of these studies looked at individuals who were dependent on opioid drugs to see if continued marijuana use led to a relapse into heroin or other opioid drugs. But in two studies that looked at how marijuana use affected the outcome for a drinking problem, it was found that marijuana use decreased the odds of achieving abstinence from alcohol or increased the chance of a relapse. As this brief review illustrates, the research is conflicting: some studies have shown that smoking marijuana did not worsen treatment outcomes, whereas other studies have shown the opposite.

TENTATIVE RECOMMENDATIONS

While everyone is different, here are some patterns I have come to see.

- For people who have struggled with alcohol and also smoked marijuana heavily, either when they drank or when not drinking, marijuana use will likely affect their ability to re- solve their alcohol problem. This is true whether their plan is abstinence from alcohol or controlled drinking. Contin- ued heavy use of marijuana will increase the chance that they relapse into excessive drinking. Using marijuana will once again likely lead to an obsession and preoccupation with using substances and will eventually negatively affect their recovery from excessive drinking.

It is time to be completely honest with yourself. If you are a heavy marijuana user and marijuana use has been a big part of your life, it probably behooves you to consider stopping. It seems likely that your marijuana use will continue to be heavy, and that could lead to excessive alcohol use again. Moreover, excessive marijuana is not good in itself. Consequently, it is my recommendation that you stop smoking it.

You may choose, however, to continue using marijuana and hoping that it does not affect your recovery from your drinking prob- lem. And it is possible you will find that it does not. As I have stressed throughout this book, you need to figure out what makes sense for you, and you need to be convinced of what you can and cannot do. If you decide to continue smoking marijuana, I offer some suggestions for you to consider in the next section.

- On the flip side, for people who have struggled with alcohol and occasionally used marijuana without it becoming a big issue in their life, a little continued marijuana use may not be detrimental to their recovery from problematic drinking.

Again, look at yourself and your relationship to marijuana. If marijuana has not been an important part of your life and you want to continue to use it infrequently, you are probably at a lower risk of marijuana hindering your recovery from your drinking problem. Read the recommendations I offer in the next section. *However, if smoking marijuana is not that important to you, you can certainly choose not to smoke it at all, just to play it safe.*

- Finally, for people who have struggled with alcohol and never smoked marijuana, staying on that path seems wise. Marijuana can be misused like alcohol, and there is no good reason to take up something new that comes with its own risks.

IF YOU DECIDE TO USE MARIJUANA

If you make the decision to continue to use marijuana, let me offer the following advice.

Begin with Abstinence

When you make the decision to stop drinking or to drink in controlled ways, I suggest that, initially, you stop smoking marijuana. See what it is like not to use marijuana as you focus on abstaining or controlling your drinking. If you never used marijuana excessively, this should be easy to do. Who knows? After not using marijuana for a while, you may even decide to give it up altogether.

For those who are heavier users of marijuana and still want to use it, I also recommend taking a break from smoking marijuana. When a person has decided to try to control alcohol use, taking a break from drinking for a month or at least a week or two can be really helpful. The same can be true for marijuana. Not using it can strengthen your confidence that you can control it, and taking a break will give you an opportunity to discover other things to do with your time. You may find that there are times when you strongly desire marijuana. This can help you understand the role that marijuana plays in your life and what you may need to do differently to manage your life without it. It is even possible that you will decide to stop using marijuana entirely, if you find that you feel better after not using it for a while.

What Is Controlled Marijuana Use?

Think about how much marijuana use makes sense for you. Will it be something you do on special occasions or something you do more regularly? And if it is more regularly, what would constitute controlled use? A few times a week? Only on the weekends? Just in the evenings? Set some guidelines and see if you can adhere to them.

Along with how often you will use it, you should also think about when it makes sense to use marijuana and when it does not. For example, some prudent guidelines would be never to smoke during work or perhaps not during the day. Or if you are taking classes, you could set a rule never to be under the influence of marijuana when in class or at times you have set aside for studying. If your marijuana use escalates, or you begin using at times when it interferes with your life, you will need to abstain from it.

Does It Increase Your Desire to Drink?

Pay attention to your thoughts and feelings if you smoke marijuana. Does it increase your desire to drink, or to drink more? Are you beginning to crave alcohol and ruminate about drinking, thus putting your sobriety or controlled use of alcohol in danger? If smoking marijuana does that to you, you need to consider that marijuana does not make sense for you, as it jeopardizes your recovery from your alcohol problem.

Does It Lead to Excessive Drinking Again?

If you find that you lapse or relapse into alcohol use, carefully look at yourself to assess if your marijuana use may have contributed to it. As I always say, being honest with yourself is most important. If using marijuana impairs your ability to resolve your drinking problem, it is clear that you need to achieve abstinence from marijuana as well.

SUMMARY

In this chapter, I discussed whether people recovering from a drinking problem can safely use marijuana. Research on this topic is limited and conflicting. While some studies have found no negative effect of marijuana use on the outcome of treatment for misusing another substance, other research has found that it can. It is my opinion that if you used marijuana excessively back when you drank excessively, and you continue to use marijuana, you run the risk of impeding or derailing the resolution of your drinking problem. On the other hand, if your use of marijuana was just occasional, continuing to use it occasionally may not affect your ability to resolve your alcohol problem.

Overall, I believe that the safest bet is not to use marijuana, but this is a decision that only you can make. If you decide to use marijuana, pay close attention to whether it influences your drinking, whether your marijuana use becomes excessive, or whether you begin to ruminate excessively about using substances. If using marijuana results in any of these three outcomes, you have proof that you shouldn't use it.

Afterword

Always bear in mind that your own resolution
to succeed is more important than any one thing.
ABRAHAM LINCOLN

In this book, I hope I have helped you understand what an alcohol problem is and how to take control of it so that you can help yourself. By using the techniques I've offered here, you may discover that you are able to help yourself and require no outside treatment. On the other hand, if you have difficulty helping yourself, I have also outlined the available treatment options.

There is no one type of treatment appropriate for everyone. Everyone is different, and these differences must be respected. Whether you resolve your drinking problem on your own or want or need some outside help is not important. Nor is how you choose to understand your drinking problem or whether you address it through abstinence or moderation. What is important is that you take control of your problem and finally do something about it.

Here are some final words of advice:

- Be honest with yourself. If you want a better life, you must acknowledge your problem with alcohol.

- Do not beat yourself up for having an alcohol problem. You are not weak. Everyone struggles with something in life, and you are no different.

- Never lose sight of your commitment to change.

- Remember the painful, troublesome consequences of your drinking. These problems are the reasons you have decided to address your drinking. Remembering them will help you stay focused on your decision. Focus will help you succeed.

- Keep in mind the vision you have and want for yourself, and remember that excessive drinking will prevent you from obtaining it and being the person you want to be.

- Work hard to create a fulfilling life for yourself without alcohol. Life can be very enjoyable, even without drinking.

- If you cannot consistently moderate your drinking, you need to accept this, move on, and work to achieve abstinence.

- There will likely be times when you will want to drink. This is normal. Despite wanting to drink, however, you can still choose not to. Urges to drink go away when you wait them out.

- Do not be seduced by reasons to drink. There are no good reasons to drink.

- It may take time to begin to feel better, but you will if you stick with your plan. Remember that returning to drinking is not the answer and will only make you feel worse in the long run.

- Never give up on yourself. You are worth the effort.

- Learn from your mistakes.

- Never stop trying. You are the only one who can get the job done.

You can do what you want to do, accomplish what you want to accomplish, attain any reasonable objective you may have in mind—not all of a sudden, perhaps not in one swift and sweeping act of achievement—but you can do it gradually, day by day and play by play, if you want to do it, if you work to do it, over a sufficiently long period of time.
WILLIAM E. HOLLER

Committing to a dream is not a one-time occurrence. It must be done daily, hourly, continually. We must choose to commit to our choice, over and over.
JOHN-ROGER AND PETER MCWILLIAMS

Bibliography

Introduction

Center for Behavioral Health Statistics and Quality. (2016, September 8). *National survey on drug use and health: Detailed tables*. Rockville, MD: Substance Abuse and Mental Health Services Administration. Retrieved from https://www.samhsa.gov

Grant, B. F., Dawson, D. A., Stinson, F. S., Chou, S. P., Dufour, M. C., & Pickering, R. P. (2004). The 12-month prevalence and trends in DSM-IV alcohol abuse and dependence: United States, 1991–1992 and 2001–2002. *Drug and Alcohol Dependence, 74*, 223–234.

Sobell, L. C., Cunningham, J. A., & Sobell, M. B. (1996). Recovery from alcohol problems with and without treatment: Prevalence in two population surveys. *American Journal of Public Health, 86*, 966–972.

Chapter 1. Do You Have a Drinking Problem?

Saunders, J. B., Assland, O. G., Babor, T. F., de la Fuente, J. R., & Grant, M. (1993). Development of the Alcohol Use Disorders Identification Test (AUDIT): WHO collaborative project on early detection of persons with harmful alcohol consumption–II. *Addiction, 88*, 791–804. Retrieved from http://dx.doi.org/10.1111/j.1360-0443.1993.tb02093.x

Seltzer, M. L. (1971). The Michigan Alcoholism Screening Test: The quest for a new diagnostic instrument. *American Journal of Psychiatry, 127*, 89–94.

Chapter 2. Why Does Drinking Cause You Difficulty?

American Society of Addiction Medicine. (1990, March–April). *ASAM News*. Retrieved from https://www.asam.org/docs/default-source/publications/1990-3-4vol5-2ocr.pdf

Armor, D. J., Polich, J. M., & Stambul, H. B. (1978). *Alcoholism and treatment*. New York, NY: John Wiley & Sons.

Davies, D. L. (1962). Normal drinking in recovered alcohol addicts. *Quarterly Journal of Studies on Alcohol, 23*, 94–104.

Dawson, D. A., Goldstein, R. B., & Grant, B. F. (2007). Rates and correlates of relapse among individuals in remission from DSM-IV alcohol dependence: A 3-year follow-up. *Alcohol Clinical and Experimental Research, 31*(12): 2036–2045.

Freud, S. (1961). *Beyond the pleasure principle* (J. Strachey, Ed. and Trans.). New York, NY: Norton. (Original work published 1920).

Goodwin, G. W. (1979). Alcoholism and heredity. *Archives of General Psychiatry, 36*, 57–61.

Heath, A. C., Madden, P. A., Bucholz, K. K., Dinwiddie, S. H., Slutske, W. S., Bierut, L. J., Rohrbaugh, J. W., Statham, D. J., Dunne, M. P., Whitfield, J. B., & Martin, N. G. (1999). Genetic differences in alcohol sensitivity and the inheritance of alcoholism risk. *Psychological Medicine, 34*, 451–453.

Jellinek, E. M. (1960). *The disease concept of alcoholism.* New Haven, CT: Hillhouse Press.

Kendell, R. E. (1965). Normal drinking by former alcohol addicts. *Journal of Studies on Alcohol, 44,* 68–83.

McLellan, A. T., Lewis, D. C., O'Brien, C. P., & Klever, H. D. (2000). Drug dependence, a chronic medical illness: Implications for treatment, insurance, and outcomes evaluation. *Journal of the American Medical Association, 284*(13), 1689–1695.

Miller, W. R., & Hester, R. K. (1980). Treating the problem drinker: Toward an informed eclecticism. In W. R. Miller (Ed.), *The addictive behaviors: Treatment of alcoholism, drug abuse, smoking, and obesity* (pp. 11–141). Elmsford, NY: Pergamon.

Miller, W. R., & Hester, R. K. (1989). Treating alcohol problems: Toward an informed eclecticism. In R. K. Hester & W. R. Miller (Eds.) *Handbook of alcoholism treatment approaches* (pp. 3–14). Elmsford, NY: Pergamon.

Mokdad, A. H., Marks, J. S., Stroup, D. G., & Gerberding, J. L. (2004). Actual causes of death in the United States, 2000. *Journal of the American Medical Association, 291*(10), 1238–1245.

National Institute on Alcohol Abuse and Alcoholism. (1992, October). The genetics of alcoholism. *Alcohol Alert,* no. 18(PH 328).

Rush, B. (1810). *Medical inquiries and observations upon the diseases of the mind.* New York, NY: Hafner.

Schuckit, M. A. (1985). Ethanol-induced changes in body sway in men at high alcoholism risk. *Archives of General Psychiatry, 43,* 375–379.

Schuckit, M. A. (1988). Reactions to alcohol in sons of alcoholics and controls. *Alcoholism: Clinical and Experimental Research, 12,* 465–470.

Schuckit, M. A., Goodwin, D. W., & Winokur, G. (1972). A half-sibling study of alcoholism. *American Journal of Psychiatry, 128,* 1132–1136.

Schuckit, M. A., & Smith, T. L. (2000). The relationships of a family history of alcohol dependence, a low level of response to alcohol and six domains of life functioning to the development of alcohol use disorders. *Journal of Studies on Alcohol, 61*(6), 827–835.

Sobell, M. B., & Sobell, L. C. (1973). Alcoholics treated by individualized behavior therapy: One year treatment outcome. *Behavior Therapy and Research, 11,* 599–618.

Sobell, M. B., & Sobell, L. C. (1976). Second year treatment outcome of alcoholics treated by individualized behavior therapy. *Behavioral Research Therapy, 14,* 195–215.

Vaillant, G. E. (1983). *The natural history of alcoholism.* Cambridge, MA: Harvard University Press.

Webster's ninth new collegiate dictionary. (1993). Springfield, MA: Merriam-Webster.

Woodward, S. B. (1838). *Essays on asylums for inebriates.* Worcester, MA.

Chapter 3. Self-Medication

Adinoff, B. (2007). Neurobiologic processes in drug reward and addiction. *Harvard Review of Psychiatry, 12,* 305–320. Retrieved from http://dx.doi.org/10.1080/10673220490910844

American Psychiatric Association. (2013). *Diagnostic and statistical manual of mental disorders* (5th ed.). Washington, DC: Author.

Frances, R. J. (1997). The wrath of grapes versus the self-medication hypothesis. *Harvard Review of Psychiatry, 4,* 287–289. Retrieved from http://dx.doi. org/10.3109/10673229709030556

Gau, S. S. F., Chong, M. Y., Yang, P., Yen, C. F., Liang, K. Y., & Cheng, A. T. A. (2007). Psychiatric and psychosocial predictors of substance use disorders among adolescents: Longitudinal study. *British Journal of Psychiatry, 190,* 42–48. Retrieved from http://dx.doi.org/10.1192/bjp.bp.106.022871

Goswami, S., Mattoo, S. K., Basu, D., & Singh, G. (2004). Substance-abusing schizophrenics: Do they self-medicate? *American Journal on Addictions, 13,* 139–150. Retrieved from http://dx.doi.org/10.1080/10550490490435795

Hall, D. H., & Queener, J. E. (2007). Self-medication hypothesis of substance use: Testing Khantzian's updated theory. *Journal of Psychoactive Drugs, 39,* 151–158. Retrieved from http://dx.doi.org/10.1080/02791072.2007.10399873

Harrington, R., Fudge, H., Rutter, M., Pickles, A., & Hill, J. (1990). Adult outcomes of childhood and adolescent depression: I. Psychiatric status. *Archives of General Psychiatry, 47,* 465–473. http://dx.doi.org/10.1001/archpsyc.1990.01810170065010

Heath, A. C. (1995). Genetic influences on alcoholism risk. *Alcohol Health & Research World, 19,* 166–171.

Henwood, B., & Padgett, D. K. (2007). Reevaluating the self-medication hypothesis among the dually diagnosed. *American Journal on Addictions, 16,* 160–165. Retrieved from http://dx.doi.org/10.1080/10550490701375368

Kessler, R. C., Berglund, P., Demler, O., Jin, R., Merikangas, K. R., & Walters, E. E. (2005). Lifetime prevalence and age-of-onset distributions of DSM-IV disorders in the National Comorbidity Survey Replication. *Archives of General Psychiatry, 62,* 593–602. Retrieved from http://dx.doi.org/10.1001/archpsyc.62.6.593

Khantzian, E. J. (1985). The self-medication hypothesis of addictive disorders: Focus on heroin and cocaine dependence. *American Journal of Psychiatry, 142,* 1259–1264. Retrieved from http://dx.doi.org/10.1176/ajp.142.11.1259

Khantzian, E. J. (1997). The self-medication hypothesis of substance use disorders: A reconsideration and recent applications. *Harvard Review of Psychiatry, 4,* 287–289. Retrieved from http://dx.doi.org/10.3109/10673229709030550

Khantzian, E. J. (1999). *Treating addiction as a human process.* Lanham, MD: Rowman & Littlefield.

Koob, G. F., & Le Moal, M. (2001). Drug addiction, dysregulation of reward, and allostasis. *Neuropsychopharmacology, 24,* 97–129. Retrieved from http://dx.doi.org /10.1016/S0893-133X(00)00195-0

Levy, M. S. (2008). Listening to our clients: The prevention of relapse. *Journal of Psychoactive Drugs, 40,* 167–172. Retrieved from http://dx.doi.org/10.1080 /02791072.2008.10400627

Lo, C. C., Cheng, T. C., & de la Rosa, I. A. (2015). Depression and substance use: A temporal-ordered model. *Substance Use and Misuse, 50,* 1274–1283. Retrieved from http://dx.doi.org/10.3109/10826084.2014.998236

National Institute on Drug Abuse. (2016). The science of substance abuse and addiction: The basics. Media guide. Retrieved from https://drugabuse.gov/publications /media-guide

Rao, U., Ryan, N. D., Birmaher, B., Dahl, R. E., Williamson, D. E., Kaufman, R. R., & Nelson, B. (1995). Unipolar depression in adolescents: Clinical outcome in adulthood. *Journal of the American Academy of Child and Adolescent Psychiatry, 34,* 566–587. Retrieved from http://dx.doi.org/10.1097/00004583-199505000-00009

Schuckit, M. A. (1994). Low level of response to alcohol as a predictor of future alcoholism. *American Journal of Psychiatry, 151,* 184–189. Retrieved from http://dx .doi.org/10.1176/ajp.151.2.184

Schuckit, M. A., & Smith, T. L. (1996). An 8-year follow-up of 450 sons of alcoholic and control subjects. *Archives of General Psychiatry, 53,* 202–210. Retrieved from http://dx.doi.org/10.1001/archpsyc.1996.01830030020005

Schuckit, M. A., Tsuang, J. W., Anthenelli, R. M., Tipp, J. E., & Nurnberger, J. I. (1996). Alcohol challenges in young men from alcoholic pedigrees and control families: A report from the COGA project. *Journal of Studies on Alcohol, 57,* 368–377. Retrieved from http://dx.doi.org/10.15288/jsa.1996.57.368

Vaillant, G. E. (1983). *The natural history of alcoholism.* Cambridge, MA: Harvard University Press.

Weiss, R. D., Griffin, M. L., & Mirin, S. M. (1992). Drug abuse as self-medication for depression: An empirical study. *American Journal of Drug and Alcohol Abuse, 18,* 121–129. Retrieved from http://dx.doi.org/10.3109/00952999208992825

Wilens, T. E., Martelon, M., Joshi, G., Bateman, C., Fried, R., Petty, C., & Biederman, J. (2011). Does ADHD predict substance-use disorders? A 10-year follow-up study of young adults with ADHD. *Journal of the American Academy of Child and Adolescent Psychiatry, 50,* 543–553. Retrieved from http://dx.doi.org/10.1016/j.jaac.2011.01.021

Wilkinson, S. L., Halpern, C. T., & Herring, A. H. (2016). Directions of the relationship between substance use and depressive symptoms from adolescence to young adulthood. *Addictive Behaviors, 60,* 64–70. Retrieved from http://dx.doi.org/10.1016 /j.addbeh.2016.03.036

Chapter 4. Getting Ready and Staying Motivated

Seligman, M. E. P., Mater, S. F., & Geer, J. H. (1968). Alleviation of learned helplessness in the dog. *Journal of Abnormal Psychology, 73,* 256–262.

Chapter 5. Can You Really Help Yourself?

American Psychiatric Association. (2013). *Diagnostic and statistical manual of mental disorders* (5th ed.). Washington, DC: Author.

Dawson, D. A. (1996). Correlates of past-year status among treated and untreated persons with former alcohol dependence: United States, 1992. *Alcoholism: Clinical and Experimental Research, 20,* 771–779.

Dupont, R. L. (1983). Foreword. In G. R. Ross (Ed.), *Treating adolescent substance abuse.* Boston: Allyn and Bacon.

Hubble, M. A., Duncan, B. L., & Miller, S. D. (1990). *The heart and soul of change.* Washington, DC: American Psychological Association.

Institute of Medicine. (1990). *Broadening the base of treatment for alcohol problems.* Washington, DC: National Academies Press.

Sobell, L. C., Cunningham, J. A., & Sobell, M. B. (1995). Recovery from alcohol problems with and without treatment: Prevalence in two population surveys. *American Journal of Public Health, 86,* 966–972.

Vaillant, G. E. (1983). *The natural history of alcoholism.* Cambridge, MA: Harvard University Press.

Chapter 6. You May Need Medical Help

Fink, E. B., Longabaugh, R., McCrady, B. M., Stout, R. L., Beattie, M., Ruggieri-Authelet, A., & McNeil, D. (1985). Effectiveness of alcoholism treatment in partial versus inpatient settings: Twenty-four month outcomes. *Addictive Behaviors, 10,* 235–48.

Chapter 7. What to Do: Abstinence or Moderation?

Dawson, D. A. (1996). Correlates of past-year status among treated and untreated persons with former alcohol dependence: United States, 1992. *Alcoholism: Clinical and Experimental Research, 20,* 771–779.

Sobell, L. C., Cunningham, J. A., & Sobell, M. B. (1996). Recovery from alcohol problems with and without treatment: Prevalence in two population surveys. *American Journal of Public Health, 86,* 966–972.

Vaillant, G. E. (1983). *The natural history of alcoholism.* Cambridge, MA: Harvard University Press.

Chapter 9. Your Personal Moderate Drinking Contract

Dawson, D. A., Grant, B., & Li, T. K. (2005). Quantifying the risks associated with exceeding recommended drinking limits. *Alcoholism: Clinical and Experimental Research, 29,* 902–908.

National Institute on Alcohol Abuse and Alcoholism. (1992, April). *Alcohol Alert,* no. 16(PH 315).

World Health Organization, Department of Mental Health and Substance Dependence. (2000). *International guide for monitoring alcohol consumption and related harm.* Geneva: Author.

Chapter 11. Managing Your Thoughts to Quit Drinking

National Institute on Alcohol Abuse and Alcoholism. (2008, October). *Helping patients who drink too much: A clinician's guide.* Bethesda, MD: Author. Excerpt retrieved from https://pubs.niaaa.nih.gov/publications/Practitioner/Clinicians Guide2005/PrescribingMeds.pdf

Chapter 12. What You Must Do to Quit Drinking

Infante, J. R., Peran, F., Martinez, M., Roldan, A., Poyatos, R., Ruiz, C., Samaniego, F., & Garrido, F. (1998). ACTH and β-endorphin in transcendental meditation. *Physiology & Behavior, 64*(3), 311–315.

Yeung, R. (1996). The acute effects of exercise on mood state. *Journal of Psychosomatic Research, 40*, 123–141.

Chapter 13. Managing Urges to Use

National Institute on Alcohol Abuse and Alcoholism. (1993, October). *Alcohol Alert*, no. 22(PH 346).

Chapter 14. Slips and Falls on the Path to Sobriety

Levy, M. (2001). Building a system to prevent relapse. *Behavioral Health Tomorrow, 10*, 34–37.

Chapter 16. Self-Help Groups and Apps

Alcoholics Anonymous. (2001). *Alcoholics Anonymous* (4th ed.). New York: Author. (Original work published 1939).

Christopher, J. (1988). *How to stay sober: Recovery without religion.* Amherst, NY: Prometheus Books.

Christopher, J. (1989). *Unhooked: Staying sober and drug free.* Amherst, NY: Prometheus Books: 1989.

Christopher, J. (1992). *SOS sobriety: The proven alternative to 12-step programs.* Amherst, NY: Prometheus Books.

Ellis, A., & Grieger, R. (1986). *Handbook of rational-emotive therapy* (Vol. 2). New York: Springer.

Kirkpatrick, J. (1986). *Goodbye hangovers, hello life: Self-help for women.* New York: Atheneum.

Kirkpatrick, J. (1990). *Turnabout: New help for women alcoholics.* New York: Bantam.

Kishline, A. (1994). *Moderate drinking: The moderation management guide for people who want to reduce their drinking.* New York: Crown Trade Paperbacks.

Levin, N. (2014). *Refuge recovery: A Buddhist path to recovery from addiction.* San Francisco: HarperOne.

SMART recovery handbook (3rd ed.). (2013). Mentor, OH: Author. [Organization's website: www.smartrecovery.org].

Trimpey, J. (1996). *Rational recovery: The new cure for substance addiction.* New York: Pocket Books.

Wilson, B. [Bill W.] (1981). *Twelve steps and twelve traditions.* New York: AA Grapevine and Alcoholics Anonymous World Services. (Original work published 1952).

Chapter 18. Medications

Anton, R. F., O'Malley, S. S., Ciraulo, D. A., Cisler, R. A., Couper, D., Donovan, D. M., Gastfriend, D. R., Hosking, J. D., Johnson, B. A., LoCastro, J. S., Longabaugh, R., Mason, J., Mattson, M. E., Miller, W. R., Pettinati, H. M., Randall, L., Swift, R.,

Weiss, R. D., Williams, L. D., & Zweben, A. (2006). Combined pharmacotherapies and behavioral interventions for alcohol dependence: The COMBINE study, a randomized controlled trial. *Journal of the American Medical Association, 295,* 2003–2017.

Besson, J., Aeby, F., Kasas, A., Lehert, P., & Potgieter, A. (1998). Combined efficacy of acamprosate and disulfiram in the treatment of alcoholism: A controlled study. *Alcoholism: Clinical and Experimental Research, 22,* 573–579.

Erwin, B. L., & Slaton, R. M. (2014). Varenicline in the treatment of alcohol use disorders. *Annals of Pharmacotherapy, 48*(11), 1445–1455. doi:10.1177/1060028014545806

Guglielmo, R., Martinotti, G., Quatrale, M., Ioime, L., Kadilli, I., Di Nicola, M., & Janiri, L. (2015). Topiramate in alcohol use disorders: Review and update. *CNS Drugs, 29*(5), 383–395. doi:10.1007/s40263-015-0244-0

Mann, K., Lehert, P., & Morgan, M. Y. (2004). The efficacy of acamprosate in the maintenance of abstinence in alcohol-dependent individuals: Results of a meta-analysis. *Alcoholism: Clinical and Experimental Research, 28,* 51–63.

Mason, B. J., Quello, S., Goodell, V., Shadan, F., Kyle, M., & Begovic, A. (2014). Gabapentin treatment for alcohol dependence: A randomized controlled trial. *JAMA Internal Medicine, 174*(1), 70–77. doi:10.1001/jamainternmed.2013.11950

Mitchell, J. M., Teague, C. H., Kayser, A. S., Bartlett, S. E., & Fields, H. L. (2012). Varenicline decreases alcohol consumption in heavy-drinking smokers. *Psychopharmacology, 223*(3), 299–306. doi:10.1007/s00213-012-2717-x

O'Malley, S. S., Jaffe, A. J., Chang, G., Schottenfeld, R. S., Meyer, R. E., & Rounsaville, B. (1992). Naltrexone and coping skills therapy for alcohol dependence. *Archives of General Psychiatry, 49,* 881–887.

Petrakis, I. L., Polig, P., Levinson, C., Nich, C., Carroll, K., & Rounsaville, B. (2005). Naltrexone and disulfiram in patients with alcohol dependence and comorbid psychiatric disorders. *Biological Psychiatry, 57,* 1128–1137.

Regier, D. A., Farmer, M. E., Rae, M. S., Locke, B. Z., Keith, S. J., Judd, L. L., & Goodwin, F. K. (1990). Comorbidity of mental disorders with alcohol and other drug abuse: Results from the Epidemiologic Catchment Area (ECA) Study. *Journal of the American Medical Association, 264,* 2511–2518.

Sovka, M., & Muller, C. A. (2017). Pharmacotherapy of alcoholism—an update on approved and off-label medications. *Expert Opinion on Pharmacotherapy, 18*(12), 1187–1199. doi:10.1080/14656566.2017.1349098

Volpicelli, J. R., Alterman, A. I., Hayashida, M., & O'Brien, C. P. (1992). Naltrexone in the treatment of alcohol dependence. *Archives of General Psychiatry, 49,* 876–880.

Volpicelli, J. R., Clay, K. L., Watson, N. T., & Volpicelli, L. A. (1995). Naltrexone and the treatment of alcohol dependence. *Alcohol Health and Research World, 18,* 272–278.

Chapter 19. Can You Smoke Marijuana?

Aharonovich, E., Liu, X., Samet, S., Nunes, E., Waxman, R., & Hasin, D. (2005). Postdischarge cannabis use and its relationship to cocaine, alcohol, and heroin use: A prospective study. *American Journal of Psychiatry, 162* (8): 1507–1514. Retrieved from http://dx.doi.org/10.1176/appi.ajp.162.8.1507

Budney, A. J., Bickel, W. K., & Amass, L. (1998). Marijuana use and treatment outcome among opioid-dependent patients. *Addiction, 93*(4), 493–503. Retrieved from http://dx.doi.org/10.1046/j.1360-0443.1998.9344935.x

Budney, A. J., Higgins, S. T., & Wong, C. J. (1996). Marijuana use and treatment outcome in cocaine-dependent patients. *Experimental and Clinical Psychopharmacology, 4*(4), 396–403. Retrieved from http://dx.doi.org/10.1037/1064-1297.4.4.396

Drug Enforcement Administration. (n.d.). Cannabis, coca, and poppy: Nature's addictive plants. Retrieved from https://www.deamuseum.org/ccp/opium/history.html

Epstein, D. H., & Preston, K. L. (2003). Does cannabis use predict poor outcome for heroin-dependent patients on maintenance treatment? Past findings and more evidence against. *Addiction, 98*(3), 269–279. Retrieved from http://dx.doi.org/10.1046/j.1360-0443.2003.00310.x

Foundation for a Drug-Free World. (2020). Alcohol: A short history. Retrieved from https://www.drugfreeworld.org/drugfacts/alcohol/a-short-history.html

Hill, K. P., Bennett, H. E., Griffin, M. L., Connery, H. S., Fitzmaurice, G. M., Subramaniam, G., Woody, G. E., & Weiss, R. D. (2013). Association of cannabis use with opioid outcomes among opioid-dependent youth. *Drug and Alcohol Dependence, 132*(1–2), 342–345. Retrieved from http://dx.doi.org/10.1016/j.drugalcdep.2013.02.030

Labigalini, E., Jr., Rodrigues, L. R., & Da Silveria, D. X. (1999). Therapeutic use of cannabis by crack addicts in Brazil. *Journal of Psychoactive Drugs, 31*(4): 451–455. Retrieved from http://dx.doi.org/10.1080/02791072.1999.10471776

Lawler, A. (2019, June 12). Oldest evidence of marijuana use discovered in 2500-year-old cemetery in peaks of western China. *Science*. doi:10.1126/science.aay3693

Mojarrad, M., Samet, J. H., Cheng, D. M., Winter, M. R., & Saitz, R. (2014). Marijuana use and achievement of abstinence from alcohol and other drugs among people with substance dependence: A prospective cohort study. *Drug and Alcohol Dependence, 142*, 91–97. Retrieved from http://dx.doi.org/10.1016/j.drugalcdep.2014.06.006

Nirenberg, T. D., Cellucci, T., Liepman, M. R., Swift, R. M., & Sirota, A. D. (1996). Cannabis versus other illicit drug use among methadone maintenance patients. *Psychology of Addictive Behaviors, 10*(4), 222–227. doi:10.1037/0893-164X.10.4.222

Saxon, A. J., Calsyn, D. A., Greenberg, D., Blaes, P., Haver, V. M., & Stanton, V. (1993). Urine screening for marijuana among methadone-maintained patients. *American Journal on Addictions, 2*(3): 207–211. Retrieved from http://dx.doi.org/10.3109/10550499309113940

Wasserman, D. A., Weinstein, M. G., Havassy, B. E., & Hall, S. M. (1998). Factors associated with lapses to heroin during methadone maintenance. *Drug and Alcohol Dependence, 52*(3), 183–192. Retrieved from http://dx.doi.org/10.1016/S0376-8716(98)00092-1

Index

ABCs, of overcoming addictions, 225
abstinence, 35, 156–57, 165–68; indications for, 100–101; marijuana effects on, 267–76; moderation vs., 7, 10, 44–45, 95–102, 147–50; as number one priority, 157–58, 162–63, 168, 176, 178, 194, 223; as only option, 1, 35, 139, 142, 148–50, 214, 224, 228; thought patterns for, 155–68; trial periods, 43, 110–11, 146–47. *See also* quitting drinking
acamprosate (Campral), 252–53, 257–58
acetaldehyde dehydrogenase, 254
addiction, 54, 79, 182; effect on the brain, 52; overcoming, 225; vulnerability to, 31–32
addictive voice recognition technique (AVRT), 230
alcohol abuse, 34
alcohol consumption, inability to control. *See* loss of control
alcohol counselors, 155, 210, 236
alcohol dehydrogenase, 254
alcohol dependence, 34, 259
alcohol-free activities: for abstinence, 172–73, 187–88; for moderation, 110, 111, 113, 120, 122, 124; for quitting/sobriety, 157–58, 169–270, 171–72, 175, 199, 205
alcoholic beverages: alcohol content, 107, 119; avoidance of certain types, 118–19, 142, 143. *See also* beer; hard liquor; wine
"alcoholic" label, 2, 29, 30
Alcoholics Anonymous (AA), 1, 35, 86, 230–31; abstinence-only philosophy, 96, 214; meetings, 1, 2, 4, 171, 177–78, 216, 218–20, 224; one-day-at-a-time philosophy, 159–60, 204, 216; program and Twelve Steps, 216–19, 220

alcoholism, 1, 2–3, 4, 6, 41–42; historical perspectives, 34–36; as personal weakness, 29–32
alcohol problem: admission of, 4, 63; ambivalence about, 64–68, 73, 76; causes, 9, 29–48; downplaying of, 163; duration, 97, 99; self-appraisal of, 8–9, 15–28, 29–32
alcohol use: as coping mechanism, 32, 156, 185, 186; duration, 100; historical perspective, 267; justification for, 167–68; prevalence, 156–57; pros and cons, 64, 67–72, 163, 164; quantity vs. quality, 20. *See also* drinking frequency; drinking limits
alcohol use disorders, 7–8, 34; continuum of severity, 34, 96, 212, 213, 221, 268–69
Alcohol Use Disorders Identification Test (AUDIT), 21, 24–26
altered consciousness, 267–69
ambivalence, 64–68, 73, 76
American Hospital Association, 33
American Medical Association, 33
American Psychiatric Association, 33, 80
American Society of Addiction Medicine (ASAM), 33, 36
anger, 18, 122, 125, 185, 204, 238, 240
Antabuse (disulfiram), 252–55
anxiety, 49–50, 51, 53–54, 89, 167, 199, 206, 260
apps, for substance use problems, 231–32, 233
assertiveness training, 204, 240
attitude: in intoxication, 20; irrational, 225; right, 84–85, 86, 88, 205, 225

bars: alcohol-free, 178; drinking at, 106–7, 112, 121, 123, 138–39, 149–50, 270